Teenagers' Citizenship

Young teenagers in Britain today are commonly portrayed in a negative light. At best, they are regarded as apathetic and at worst, as a threat to civil society. But can citizenship education overcome teenage apathy or are teenagers engaged in new or alternative forms of participation?

Intended to tackle political disaffection amongst the young, the introduction of compulsory citizenship education into the National Curriculum has generated a plethora of new interests in the politics of childhood and youth. *Teenagers' Citizenship* explores teenagers' acts of and engagement with citizenship and examines the role of citizenship education in creating future responsible citizens. Through extracts from interviews, diaries, internet and radio-based discussions and photography, it presents teenagers' own perspectives on their exclusion from participation, their experiences of statutory citizenship education and their own acts of citizenship and civic engagement.

Teenagers' Citizenship moves beyond viewing those under the age of eighteen as 'citizens-in-the-making', by demonstrating the ways many teenagers are involved as active citizens in their schools and communities. It will be of interest to policy-makers and academics working in the fields of youth and citizenship, as well as students of education, human geography, politics, sociology and social policy.

Susie Weller is a Research Fellow in the Families & Social Capital ESRC Research Group, London South Bank University, UK.

Relationships & resources
Series editors: Janet Holland and Rosalind Edwards
London South Bank University

A key contemporary political and intellectual issue is the link between the relationships that people have and the resources to which they have access. When people share a sense of identity, hold similar values, trust each other and reciprocally do things for each other, this has an impact on the social, political and economic cohesion of the society in which they live. So, are changes in contemporary society leading to deterioration in the link between relationships and resources, or new and innovative forms of linking, or merely the reproduction of enduring inequalities? Consideration of relationships and resources raises key theoretical and empirical issues around change and continuity over time as well as time use, the consequences of globalization and individualization for intimate and broader social relations, and location and space in terms of communities and neighbourhoods. The books in the series are concerned with elaborating these issues and will form a body of work that will contribute to academic and political debate.

Other titles include:

Moving On
Bren Neale and Jennifer Flowerdew

Sibling Identity and Relationships
Sisters and brothers
Rosalind Edwards, Lucy Hadfield, Helen Laucey and Melanie Mauthner

Teenagers' Citizenship

Experiences and education

Susie Weller

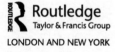

Routledge
Taylor & Francis Group

LONDON AND NEW YORK

First published 2007
by Routledge
2 Park Square, Milton Park, Abingdon, Oxon OX14 4RN

Simultaneously published in the USA and Canada
by Routledge
711 Third Avenue, New York, NY 10017

Routledge is an imprint of the Taylor & Francis Group, an informa business

© 2007 Susie Weller

Typeset in Sabon by
GreenGate Publishing Services, Tonbridge, Kent

British Library Cataloguing in Publication Data
A catalogue record for this book is available from the British Library

Library of Congress Cataloging in Publication Data
Weller, Susie.
   Teenagers' citizenship : experiences and education / Susie Weller.
      p. cm. – (Relationships and resources)
   Includes bibliographical references and index.
   ISBN 978-0-415-40463-1 (hardback) – ISBN 978-0-415-40464-8 (pbk.)
1. Teenagers—Great Britain—Attitudes. 2. Citizenship—Study and
teaching—Great Britain. 3. Social participation—Great Britain. 4. Young volunteers—Great Britain. 5. Communitarianism—Great Britain. I. Title.
   HQ799.G7W38 2007
   323.60835'0941—dc22
   2006036671

ISBN10: 0–415–40463–0 (hbk)
ISBN10: 0–415–40464–9 (pbk)
ISBN13: 978–0–415–40463–1 (hbk)
ISBN13: 978–0–415–40464–8 (pbk)

Contents

Illustrations

Plates

Tables

Acknowledgements

With thanks to Prof. Ros Edwards and Prof. Janet Holland, series editors, for all their support and help with this book. I would like to thank my PhD supervisors, Dr. Fiona Smith and Dr. Nicola Ansell, in the Department of Geography and Earth Sciences at Brunel University, for all their contributions. I would also like to thank Dr. Jon Binnie and Dr. Warwick Murray for their support and interest during the early stages of this research.

I would especially like to thank Roger, Steve, Tina and all the other members of staff at the case study school for their enthusiasm, help and for allowing me a great deal of access to and time within the school. I would particularly like to thank Roger and Steve for the geographical inspiration they instilled in me as a pupil.

My gratitude also goes to a vast number of people on the Isle of Wight who contributed to and aided this research. I would especially like to thank all those at Isle of Wight Radio who made the children and teenagers' phone-in possible; all those who participated in radio and web board discussions; all the teenagers at the case study school who completed questionnaire surveys. I reserve my utmost respect and gratitude for Agnuz, Bob, Bob Stevens, Chloe, Crateser, Duey, Funda, Gumdrop, Janna, Kat, Katie, Kaz, Kendal, Kimbo, Kitty Sandoral, Lee, Loki, Matt, Nikki, Rammstein Nut and Tommey. I would particularly like to thank them for never (openly) saying 'oh no she's back again, hasn't she finished that project yet?'; for their sustained enthusiasm and interest; and for providing me with a window into their lives, frustrations and creativity.

For their financial support I would like to thank the Department of Geography and Earth Sciences at Brunel University. I am also grateful to the trustees of the 'Newport Grammar School Charity' and the 'Godshill Grammar School Endowment Foundation' on the Isle of Wight who provided financial support during my doctoral research.

For their invaluable support as fellow research students I would like to thank Dr. Thomas Dewez, Pedro Costas, Dr. Phill Teasdale and Dr. Leo Zeilig. I would especially like to thank Dr. John Barker for the tea, chats and a highly valued friendship that got me through the research process and beyond.

My greatest appreciation is reserved for my family – for my parents' continuous support; for their practical help, emotional guidance and for all my childhood experiences on the Island. I would also like to thank Calum and Holly for their invaluable role as research assistants in the design and implementation of this research. Finally, I would like to thank Rob, for his unconditional support and help through all the highs and lows; for his encouragement, motivation and amazing enthusiasm in the face of adversity!

Abbreviations and acronyms

ASBO	Anti-Social Behaviour Order
CYPU	Children and Young People's Unit
DfEE	Department for Education and Employment
DfES	Department for Education and Skills
EU	European Union
NfER	National Foundation for Educational Research
NGO	Non-Governmental Organization
NSPCC	National Society for the Prevention of Cruelty to Children
NSSC	New Social Studies of Childhood
OFSTED	Office for Standards in Education
QCA	Qualifications and Curriculum Authority
UNCRC	United Nations Convention on the Rights of the Child

Chapter 1

Introduction
On being a teenager

Setting the scene

Citizenship or civics education has a more established foundation in many European countries and in the USA than in Britain. Several studies have sought to make international comparisons between the provision and implementation of citizenship education (Hahn, 1999; Kerr, 1999a; 1999b; Nelson and Kerr, 2005; Osler, 2005). The approach taken by different nations may be placed on a continuum with those embedded in a more communitarian or civic republican tradition, placing more emphasis on the importance of such education than those from more liberal perspectives (Osler and Starkey, 2005a). Context and tradition are vital to understanding the focus of citizenship education in different countries. In France, for example, the emphasis is upon civic knowledge, whilst in Sweden the key focus is on values-based education (Nelson and Kerr, 2005). Context also changes over time. For example, within England there has been a move away from the Conservative Government's more liberal understanding of active citizenship and self-help in the 1980s and early 1990s, towards a vision of citizenship based upon liberal communitarianism and democratic renewal under the current New Labour Government (Gifford, 2004; Nelson and Kerr, 2005). What constitutes citizenship is, however, complex.

In September 2002 citizenship education became a compulsory element of the secondary school curriculum in England. With focus on the development of *future responsible citizens* the subject was formalized in order to challenge voter apathy, counter alienation, promote *active* citizenship and provide a unifying element to the government's policy on social exclusion. Policy-makers' adherence to *active* citizenship was challenged six months later when in March 2003 several million people took to the streets in protest against military action in Iraq (Weller, 2006a). What was both unique and significant about several of these campaigns was that they were organized and implemented by, and for, children and teenagers of compulsory school age (Weller, 2006a). Abandoning their classrooms, but often not their school uniforms, young people from many cultural backgrounds joined in solidarity with their counterparts across the world, challenging the notion of teenage apathy (Bedell, 2003). Campaigners gathered in diverse places from rural Cornwall to Parliament Square in London, often disregarding the conventional rules of protest by sitting in the streets, symbolically chanting 'this is what democracy looks like' (Walker, 2003). The events were hugely controversial, with educational authorities and schools, citing their duty of care to parents, threatening participants with punishments associated with truancy (see also Cunningham and Lavalette, 2004). As childhood is principally upheld as a time of education and development (Holloway and Valentine, 2000a), it is perhaps not surprising that many felt school was the more appropriate place for children and teenagers to learn politics. Phipps (2003) suggests that these protests signal the emergence of a 'new kind of political protester', whose voice has, for so long, been neglected particularly beyond the realms of the classroom. Against dominant discourses which suggest that teenagers are apathetic such actions illustrate how the young *are* interested and involved in affairs commonly deemed part of the adult world (Phipps, 2003).

The overriding aim of this book is to explore teenagers' acts of and engagement with citizenship. It draws upon a three-year study,[1] undertaken during the introduction of compulsory citizenship education, which examined teenagers' exclusion from local governance in rural areas; the influence of citizenship education on the political actions of teenagers; and the extent to which teenagers shape their local areas through their own interpretations and acts of citizenship. In the study social exclusion was used in a broad sense to reflect exclusion from civil and political aspects of citizenship. In these terms all those under the age of eighteen may be seen as excluded from discussions on and engagement with conventional understandings of citizenship, as those under eighteen are constructed as 'citizens-in-the-making'.

Overwhelmingly the book seeks to promote teenagers' voices and experiences. It is not an evaluation of citizenship education per se, although many of the findings presented do have very real policy implications. Rather it is an exploration of the understandings and experiences of teenagers in relation to active citizenship. As later chapters reveal, the age-based status that teenagers are afforded in such lessons has significant impacts on their engagement with the subject. Furthermore, the study set out to examine the role that citizenship education could play in engaging teenagers in their local communities. The inversion of this enquiry was revealed during the course of the research. Those already participating as active citizens were more likely to be engaged by citizenship education. This has significant implications for the challenges that the curriculum faces in involving those most disaffected, as well as illustrating the acts of citizenship in which many already participate. Indeed, many of the teenagers involved in the study highlighted numerous ways in which they contributed to their communities and engaged in practices of citizenship.

In this book I will present two key arguments which highlight teenagers' challenging relationship with citizenship, as well as demonstrating the (often unconventional) ways many teenagers are involved as active citizens. First, I call for a cumulative notion of citizenship where children, teenagers and adults alike are all represented as full citizens who, throughout their life, learn, develop and exert different forms of citizenship in different spaces. Second, I argue for a more cosmopolitan approach to teenagers' citizenship, particularly in terms of the structure of the citizenship curriculum. The book presents a more holistic approach to teenagers' lives as citizens, bringing together their experiences both inside and out of school. In doing so, teenagers' perspectives are explored in relation to participation in decision-making at school (chapter 4); participation in creative and innovative acts of citizenship outside school (chapter 5); and their inclusion within and exclusion from decision-making in the local community (chapter 6). Particular emphasis is placed upon spaces of citizenship as a means of illustrating the ways in which teenagers' engagement (re)shapes places within their school and community. Furthermore, charting the power relations inherent within those spaces highlights the challenges teenagers face to become recognized as active citizens.

This introductory chapter begins by outlining the conceptual framework underpinning the research on which this book is based before turning to provide a comprehensive introduction to the category 'teenager' and the main contexts which shape teenagers' lived experiences. Within the modern conceptualization[2] of 'childhood' children and young teenagers are excluded from the 'adult' realms of socio-political participation and citizenship by their status as non-voters. Finally, details of the research site, participants and methods adopted will be outlined. This chapter, therefore, provides the backdrop for exploring teenagers' relationship with citizenship.

Thinking about teenagers' citizenship

The study was undertaken as a geographical-based enquiry and whilst the research has drawn upon and been influenced by an eclectic group of disciplines and conceptual backgrounds, two key understandings have remained prominent. The first is the 'New Social Studies of Childhood' (NSSC) and more specifically the emergence of children's geographies (for a summary see Matthews, 2003). The second grounding for this study is 'New Feminist Perspectives on Citizenship'. Each of these perspectives is discussed below.

A geographical perspective

Whilst the study drew upon literature and research from a wide range of disciplines including sociology, politics, psychology, education and anthropology, the most significant disciplinary influence was geography.

Geographical research offers an alternative perspective on the social world by highlighting and exploring the importance of space and place (see also Massey *et al.*, 1999). In essence human geography is principally concerned with the inter-relationship between humans (and in some research non-humans) and the environment (Johnston *et al.*, 2000), thus (re)connecting 'the social' with environments, landscapes, communities and so on. These spatial spheres are not necessarily 'real' or 'out there' but encompass a myriad of manifestations, from real to imagined, from physical to abstract and from conceptual to ephemeral. Similar spaces often mean alternative things to different people, and many individuals are likely to be members of a number of communities which are not obviously tied to a specific geographical space such as a village or neighbourhood but do have important spatial manifestations.

Human geography both contributes to and draws upon many disciplines within the social sciences. In doing so, geographical research highlights the importance of viewing 'the social' as spatially constructed, as well as regarding 'the spatial' as socially constructed (Massey *et al.*, 1999). Moreover, the significance of space and place has come to the fore in contemporary social research proving fundamental in understanding the social world (Allen *et al.*, 1999; Gordon *et al.*, 2000). In these terms many geographers view, explore, research and analyse the world and society using their geographical imaginations (see Johnston *et al.*, 2000: 298–301), and so it is with such a geographical perspective in mind that this book progresses through an exploration of teenagers' relationship with citizenship. The spatial will be highlighted as a significant feature of teenagers' engagement as citizens and indeed that 'geography matters' (see Massey *et al.*, 1999). For example, schools, the formal arena for citizenship education, are social and political spaces, which Gordon *et al.* (2000) describe as consisting of a number of layers including the official, the informal and the physical.

Despite the trend in human geography and other social sciences towards the consideration of inequalities and marginalized 'others', children have not featured highly on research agendas until relatively recently (James, 1990). Whilst work in the early 1970s did begin to focus on children's use and experience of place and space (Blaut and Stea, 1971; Bunge, 1973), Bunge's (1973) early recognitions of children as the largest minority group were largely neglected until around a decade later. Emerging as an ontological response to the dominance of adult-centred studies inherent in the academy, this area of work:

> focuses on how children's perceptions, experiences and opportunities are socially and spatially structured, and which examines the reproduction of culture and social life through children.
>
> (Johnston *et al.*, 2000: 78)

Geographical research *with* and *on* children has developed along two lines of enquiry. The first draws upon psychology; for example, work on children's environmental behaviour and the influence of cognitive development upon children's conceptions of space (Piche, 1981; Hart, 1984; Matthews, 1992; Philo, 1997; Holloway and Valentine, 2000a). In contrast, the second approach takes a more sociological stance and has been concerned with agency and children's spatial experiences, regarding young people as competent social actors (Philo, 1997; Holloway and Valentine, 2000a).

Rallied by James's (1990) influential paper 'Is there a "place" for children in geography?', geographical research with children has gathered momentum since the mid 1990s, becoming a vibrant, influential and growing body of work (see, for example, Matthews, 2003 for a summary). Popular focus has moved towards the greater recognition of children as social actors (Piche, 1981). Feminist, post-structural and post-modern approaches have all been influential in the development of contemporary children's geographies, placing more emphasis on 'otherness', diversity and difference (Hill and Michelson, 1981; Sibley, 1991). This work has seen the development of a dedicated academic journal *Children's Geographies* and numerous conferences dedicated to research with the young. Geographers have placed children's needs on research and policy agendas by drawing attention to the diverse experiences of children and young people across the globe (Weller, 2006b). Many have also been at the forefront of promoting alternative ways of conducting research *with* young people (see, for example, Matthews *et al.*, 1998a; Valentine, 1999; Matthews, 2001; Young and Barrett, 2001; Leyshon, 2002; Barker and Weller, 2003a; 2003b). Space and place, as will be illustrated throughout this book, are highly relevant to teenagers' acts of citizenship.

Whilst the work of children's geographers and other children-centred researchers has been invaluable in placing the needs and experiences of children and young people on research and policy agendas within the UK, there has been little focus explicitly on teenagers' lives (with the exceptions of Sibley, 1995; Matthews *et al.*, 2000a; Skelton, 2000; Tucker and Matthews, 2001; Tucker, 2003). Skelton (2000) provides one of the most detailed discussions of the neglect of teenagers in geography to date, and draws upon her own research exploring the leisure-time experiences of teenage girls in Wales, UK, to remedy this. Matthews *et al.* (1998b) also argue that the use of spaces by young teenagers has rarely been documented and set out to resolve this by exploring their micro-geographies. Furthermore, Valentine (2004) discusses teenagers' use of and treatment in public space, whilst Tucker (2003) has explicitly drawn attention to the experiences of teenage girls and their use of recreational spaces in areas of rural Britain (see also Tucker and Matthews, 2001). Tucker's analysis draws upon the notion of 'generation' to explore how children are defined in relation to adults, in addition to notions of sameness and diversity within and between generations (Tucker, 2003).

We have to cross the Atlantic to the USA, however, to find more explicit focus on teenagers in the work of, for example, Cahill (2000), Aitken (2001) and Mattingly (2001).

A 'children-centred' approach

Akin to the development of children's geographies, research with children and young people within the broader social sciences has gathered momentum in the past two decades. The direction of this work has developed in response to a number of major criticisms of previous studies *on* children. First, positivist research with its focus on measurement and assessment, and treatment of children as research objects rather than research subjects has been criticized (Barker and Weller, 2003b). Second, children's experiences were often problematically subsumed within other aspects of study such as 'education' or 'the family' rather than placing value on their own views (Barker and Weller, 2003b). The final criticism of children's place in the research world was that children were not regarded as human beings, but rather as human becomings who would assume competency and 'completeness' on entering adulthood (James *et al.*, 1998; Muscroft, 1999; Holloway and Valentine, 2000b). There are many parallels between the emergence of research *with* children and the development of feminist research exploring gender. As women's studies aimed to deconstruct patriarchal theory, children's studies aimed to counter 'adultism' (Alanen, 1994). As a result, an increasingly critical approach to children's experiences has been fostered, focusing on empowerment, participation and self-determination (James, 1990; Matthews and Limb, 1999). Indeed, contemporary research with children is heavily influenced by feminist, post-modern and post-structural writings.

In response to this neglect of children and young people's own experiences a growing body of multi-disciplinary work has developed and is commonly referred to as the 'New Social Studies of Childhood' (NSSC) (James *et al.*, 1998; Holloway and Valentine, 2000b). The NSSC are framed by the understanding that research should be conducted *with* and not *on* children and young people. The NSSC uphold a number of key values which seek to challenge past understandings of childhood, for example, deconstructing the notion that children are human becomings rather than human beings. The first way in which this is achieved is by identifying childhood as a social construction, both time- and place-specific (Holloway and Valentine, 2000a). This approach acknowledges the diversity in children's lives in terms of their societal backgrounds and the period in history in which they live out these experiences. Beyond this, the second means by which the NSSC challenge past conceptions is by acknowledging that children are social actors in their own right, shaping and controlling their own life worlds (Holloway and Valentine, 2000a; Morrow, 2000). This is not to say that children's agency is not controlled or limited to different extents by external factors, in much the same way as other social groups have both similar and unique controls imposed upon their lives. Fundamentally, the NSSC recognize and uphold the dictum that child-hood is not a universal category: that 'the child' does not exist. Furthermore, whilst children as a social group may have similar experi-ences, their characters are unique and differentiated by other factors such as gender, ethnicity and class. The NSSC also advocate research which acknowledges children as valuable research subjects (Holloway and Valentine, 2000a; Morrow, 2000).

In charting the research completed under the auspices of the NSSC, James *et al.* (1998) outline a fourfold typology illustrating the ways in which researchers have conceptualized 'the child/children'. The first conceptualiza-tion is 'the social structural child' where the researcher acknowledges that children's lives vary but it is contended that childhood is universal. The sec-ond way of studying children is through the lens of 'the minority group child'. This is a politicized version of the socio-structural child that con-structs children as a minority group in relation to adults (James *et al.*, 1998; Holloway and Valentine, 2000b; James and James, 2004). The third concep-tualization is 'the socially constructed child' where 'childhood' is regarded as time- and place-specific. In these terms there is no universal category of childhood (James *et al.*, 1998; Holloway and Valentine, 2000b). The final means of viewing childhood is 'the tribal child' which is a politicized version of the socially constructed child. This approach explores the differences between children and examines the way in which children view themselves and their relationships with others; children's actions exist in an almost sep-arate world to adults (James *et al.*, 1998; Holloway and Valentine, 2000b; Mayall, 2002; James and James, 2004).

Accompanying ideological shifts in children-centred research has been the move towards developing methods which reflect and value the compe-tency of children and teenagers. Contemporary children-centred research draws many parallels with participatory (action) research (see, for exam-ple, Park, 1999; Taylor, 1999; Krimerman, 2001), where researchers and participants are active collectors or 'co-producers' of data (Alderson, 2000a; Kellet, 2005). Participatory methods are more transparent and less invasive than conventional ethnographies, allowing participants to take an active role within the research process (O'Kane, 2000). Contemporary children-centred research utilizes techniques which recog-nize the diverse ways that children and teenagers communicate (Thomas and O'Kane, 1999; Barker and Weller, 2003a; 2003b). Such methods expand upon written and oral techniques, to incorporate, for example, drawing, photography, stories or song (Alderson, 1995), as well as inter-views and discussions.

A feminist approach to citizenship

The writings associated with 'New Feminist Perspectives on Citizenship' are the final key influence on the conceptual framework of this study. Definitions of citizenship will be elaborated upon in chapter 2, but it is important to note here the lessons that an analysis of teenagers' citizenship can learn from the way new feminist perspectives on citizenship deconstruct the concept in relation to women's experiences. Lister (1997a; 1997b), for example, explores women's exclusion from full citizenship and provides a comprehensive exploration of the exclusionary and inclusionary aspects of citizenship which define different groups and individuals as 'insiders' and 'outsiders'. Furthermore, Foster (1997) outlines a feminist critique of citizenship (education) suggesting that, in its current form, the concept is a patriarchal construct. In these terms the assignment of women to the private sphere renders their true access to formal (public) civic institutions problematic (Foster, 1997; Dillabough and Arnot, 2000). Again, important lessons can be drawn from both Lister's (1997b) analysis and Foster's (1997) critique, transposed onto the examination of teenagers' exclusion from citizenship. At the same time it must be remembered that, within the context of this research, (adult) women have rights to formal spaces of citizenship through political institutions such as elections, which are not extended to those under the age of eighteen.

On being a teenager

The study from which this book stems elected to focus on young teenagers for a number of reasons. First, those aged 13–16 have often been neglected in both research and policy. Valentine (2003), for example, highlights that research with children often focuses on two age groups, with children categorized as those aged 5–16, and youth comprising of those aged 16–25. Furthermore, it has been argued that the influential United Nations Convention on the Rights of the Child (UNCRC) places greatest emphasis on middle childhood (De Waal, 2002). The increasing independence of young teenagers is ultimately neglected when subsumed into such categories, for example, studies which focus on the increasing amounts of time that children in the West spend under the supervision of adults in privatized spaces, such as the home or commercial play facilities, are of little relevance to many young teenagers, who seldom discuss play-spaces or toys (Weller, 2006b). The second argument for focusing on young teenagers is that the introduction of compulsory citizenship education in secondary schools in England provides an important context to this research and so inherently includes those aged 11–16. This curriculum development has generated a plethora of interest in the politics of childhood and youth and this book examines the role of citizenship education in creating 'future responsible citizens'. Finally, teenagers are frequently represented in a negative light in both the media and policy debates. As subsequent chapters will highlight many *are* engaged in acts of citizenship which often go unrecognized.

In seeking to provide a backdrop to teenagers' engagement with citizenship it is important to outline what it means to be a teenager in contemporary Western society. This chapter now turns to exploring the 'betweenness' experienced by young teenagers by examining the constructions and influence of both 'childhood' and 'youth'.

Teenagers and 'childhood'

Teenagers' lived experiences are, in part, constructed and structured by the notion of childhood. Discourses around childhood centre principally on incompetence, dependence, vulnerability and incompleteness. Research on childhood has often been approached from a developmental standpoint. Much work in psychology, for example that of De Mausse, has focused upon children's experiences in terms of age-based competencies. This epistemological approach may be linked to Darwinian thought on evolution (Archard, 1993). Furthermore, work in psychoanalysis has drawn attention to important philosophical debates relating to personhood and the question of whether knowledge is innate at birth, as upheld in the writings of Plato and Descartes, or acquired through experiences, as suggested by, for example, Piaget and Locke (Miller, 1982; Archard, 1993). Such studies, whilst they can justifiably be accused of biological determinism, have been fundamentally important in shaping discourse surrounding concept(s) of childhood and children's capabilities and are upheld today in, for example, the structuring of schooling.

This book draws upon notions surrounding social constructivism, and considers 'childhood' as time- and place-specific (Holloway and Valentine, 2000a; Weller, 2006b). Discussion on the social construction of childhood is most eminently associated with the writings of Aries (1962). Aries' thesis proposed that no conceptualization of childhood existed in the Middle Ages. Drawing such conclusions principally from an examination of medieval art, Aries suggests that childhood is not a biological given. Interpreting the paintings of the time, he argues that children were, instead, depicted as small adults (Aries, 1962). Alternatively, the representation of children in such a form may say more about the artists of that time than the absence of childhood. Nevertheless, the conceptualization of childhood as distinct from adulthood, Aries suggests, originated from the onset of the Industrial Revolution and ultimately led to the separation of the life-worlds of adults and children. Aries' work has, however, received criticism. Archard (1993), for example, argues that 'modernity' has created a particular type of childhood, one which is particularly difficult to distinguish from a symbolic ideal. Furthermore, Martindale (1994) suggests that Aries' thesis lacks evidence, although what form of 'evidence' is not made apparent. Alternatively, Kennedy (1998) outlines the development of the modern 'adult', tracing a move from medieval collectivism to individualism from the late fifteenth century. Whilst Aries' thesis remains heavily critiqued, particularly in terms of its exaltation of the modern conceptualization as an ideal, it remains highly influential in many spheres of social science.

Despite debate which calls for the recognition of children's diverse experiences, contemporary Western childhood is, however, itself dichotomized (Valentine, 1996; Gerrard, 1999). Jenks (1996) describes the Dionysian child as a 'little devil' exhibiting inherently bad tendencies, which require control. This half of the dualism was developed during the late sixteenth and early seventeenth centuries, and has been upheld in much Christian doctrine alongside ideas of original sin (Jenks, 1996). In contrast the Apollonian child is seen as pure and innocent and in need of protection (Jenks, 1996). Such a dichotomy may be likened to Freud's 'civilised' and 'savage' children, the former signifying 'the child' as a voice of neurosis, whilst the latter represents the voice of desire (Kennedy, 2000). One element which links the Apollonian child and the Dionysian child is the notion of dependency. Children, bound by the concept of childhood, are therefore dependent upon, and dichotomized from, adults. This implicitly shapes their lived experiences in all domains of society.

Parallel to feminist writings, it is important to deconstruct research which essentializes children's experiences and refers only to 'the child'. As Gittens (1998) suggests, children are not self-defined as a social group, but have a multiplicity of identities. Stainton-Rogers and Stainton-Rogers (1992) also highlight the importance of the construction of language and narrative in the definition of 'the child'. Arguably, the construction of such discourse enforces, consciously or unconsciously, some element of identity within children as a social group upheld within the institutions of education and organized play.

Teenagers and 'youth'

Whilst on one level teenagers are positioned in relation to childhood, discourses around youth are also extremely influential. The construction and representation of 'youth' has many parallels to that of 'childhood', in that both are frequently viewed in terms of deficit: as non-adult. As Wyn and White (1997) argue, 'youth' is neither a single category nor an homogenous group within society. Nevertheless, in many fields 'youth' is still held to be a period in the life-course of 'growing up', and is inherently represented as a biological reality (Wyn and White, 1997). In policy 'youth' is often constructed to embody those aged between 13 and 25. Whilst childhood is also a period of 'growing up', 'youth' is presented as a transitory period: the final steps towards adulthood. Although biological changes do occur, these are embodied within social contexts (Wyn and White, 1997). The related concept of 'adolescence' places too much emphasis on physical bodily developments alone, neglecting the dynamics and diversity of 'youth' (Wyn and White, 1997).

The contemporary notion of 'youth' is often said to have developed after the Second World War when the transition to adulthood was marked by consumption and production (Wyn and White, 1997; Skelton and Valentine, 1998). From the 1950s onwards many young people acquired greater disposable income:

> Youth became a 'new category' of person, distinctive, usually male, and a potential threat to the stability of society.
>
> (Wyn and White, 1997: 18)

Smith *et al.* (2002) detail the notion of the 'neo-liberal youth'; a child who grows up to be autonomous and competitive in the global marketplace. Wyn and White (1997) argue that ideas of 'youth' were also apparent in the late nineteenth century when working-class young people (usually male) were seen as problematic. Furthermore, despite the linguistic absence of the term 'youth' in the seventeenth century, Wyn and White (1997) suggest that this cannot be equated to the non-existence of 'youth' as a stage in the life-course, for transitions such as marriage and leaving home still occurred. The argument that the category 'youth' did not exist in the past, because it was absent linguistically, has been critiqued for closely reflecting Karl Popper's critical rationalism, in which the principle of falsification suggests that the absence of the term 'youth' is not synonymous with the non-existence of the category. Indeed, Skelton and Valentine (1998) highlight that Aries' thesis marked out adolescence or youth as a 'breathing space' between childhood and adulthood, which began in the early eighteenth century when more wealthy 'children' were able to remain in education for longer. It is apparent, therefore, that 'youth' is an historical, social and cultural construct. This period is, Sibley suggests, one of blurred boundaries:

> adolescents are denied access to the adult world, but they attempt to distance themselves from the world of the child. At the same time they retain some links to childhood.
>
> (1995: 34–5)

'Youth' in the 1970s and 1980s was examined principally in terms of sub-culture (Wyn and White, 1997; Watt, 1998). Wyn and White (1997) critique this analysis for universalizing 'youth' into one homogenous category. Whilst there may be commonalities between many groups of young people, for example schooling, the experiences of contemporary teenagers are manifested in a multitude of ways globally. Indeed, experiences may also be radically different even within small localities (Wyn and White, 1997). The development of 'youth culture', defined by factors such as clothing and music, has led to discourse relating to juvenile delinquency, with young people seemingly contesting social norms and values. The rejection of a 'neo-liberal youth' is often equated to deviant behaviour (Smith *et al.*, 2002). Furthermore, the development of cultural studies in youth-centred research has, importantly, recognized that young people are not passive victims, but are instrumental in creating their own life-worlds, and resisting dominant cultures.

Despite much progress in youth-centred research, little work has challenged the problematic construction and use of the term 'youth'. Importantly, contemporary research, often affiliated with post-modern understandings, has sought to challenge ideas often associated with developmental psychology in order to view 'youth' as a relational problematic and to begin to explore not only difference and diversity but also power relations within and between groups of young people. Moreover, whilst groups of young people may appear to be experiencing similar circumstances, identities may be further fragmented by, for example, gender, sexuality and ethnicity (Wyn and White, 1997). 'Youth' has also come to embrace new meanings. Patterns of consumption have commodified 'youth' or 'youthfulness' as an identity to be sought after, to be purchased. 'Youth', Wyn and White (1997) suggest, has become less about 'coming of age' and more about the symbolic meanings underlying consumption. For many young people, such understandings are limited and challenged by peer pressure and socio-economic conditions. These representations of youth are, however, fundamentally important to examining teenagers' lived experiences.

Teenagers 'in-between'

Akin to the concepts of 'childhood' and 'youth' the term 'teenager' is socially and culturally constructed (Weller, 2006b). Fuelled by post-war prosperity, the emergence of the category 'teenager' in the West has often been accredited to the growth in youth consumerism and youth-oriented markets in the 1950s (Valentine *et al.*, 1998; Weller, 2006b), although there is some evidence to suggest that such a development was emerging prior to the Second World War (Miles, 2000). In these terms, and in part for the sake of marketing, 'teenager' was often represented as a positive stage, full of fun and potential for the future (Valentine *et al.*, 1998; Weller, 2006b). Such representations are juxtaposed with the often negative images of 'youth' presented in the media (Hebdige, 1988; Valentine *et al.*, 1998). More recently, however, the term 'teenager' has also been portrayed in negative ways in the media and in policy debates (Weller, 2006b). Such representations are not, however, universal and the term 'teenager' is complex and fluid, often simultaneously represented as both positive and negative (Weller, 2006b).

Participants in the research drawn on in this book did not regard themselves, nor wished to be represented, as children as they felt their increasing independence had moved them beyond the category 'child(hood)' (Weller, 2006b). As notions of growing up and maturing are seen as positives, whilst acting younger and being babyish is often viewed as negative, being labelled as a child may appear patronizing or belittling to teenagers (Weller, 2006b). At the same time, the majority refuted the idea of being referred to as 'young people' and saw this as 'cheesy' or patronizing; a term used and applied by adults not by the participants themselves (Weller, 2006b). Although a small minority preferred the phrase 'young adult', the majority advocated the term 'teenager(s)' because it represented their status in the here-and-now (Weller, 2006b). In line with the focus of children's geographies on empowerment, participants' own self-identities are, therefore, respected throughout this book.

The adult/child binary and societal constructions of childhood, adulthood and youth render teenagers, and in particular young teenagers, in a position of ambiguity. Ambiguity is essential in understanding teenagers' lived experiences (Skelton, 2000; Weller, 2006b). As Skelton (2000) suggests, those in ambiguous positions, or those who do not fit a common binary, such as adult/child or male/female, are often marginalized in Western society. The adult/child binary, whilst problematic in a number of well-documented (see Skelton, 2000) instances, is particularly challenging for teenagers as it fails to recognize their dual-positioning: simultaneously within one category whilst also being 'in-between'. A child is a young person but a young person does not necessarily have to be a child. A young person may also be an adult. At the same time a teenager may be a child, a youth or an adult or in-between any of those categories (Weller, 2006b). Matthews and Limb (1999) suggest that the terms 'children' and 'childhood', often problematically seen as synonymous, are frequently applied as 'umbrella' terms encompassing teenager, youth, young person and adolescent. Moreover, Aitken suggests that the interchangability between child, teenager and adolescent highlights their 'shifting identities ... [and] ... the baggage (and disempowerment)' (2001: 7) encapsulated in different definitions. Each term carries with it a set of assumptions and depictions or 'baggage'. Reflecting the feelings of many participants in this research, Sibley (1995) highlights the 'fuzziness' of boundaries, illustrating how teenagers or adolescents transverse the categories of childhood and adulthood, whilst at the same time distancing themselves from both categories (Weller, 2006b). Whilst teenagers are often active agents in this movement or distancing, they are nevertheless ultimately positioned as 'in-between' (Weller, 2006b).

The ambiguity of teenagers' positioning is reinforced in UK legislation and policy where an unclear distinction between childhood and adulthood exists (Weller, 2006b). Instead the process is more fluid. A person is, for example, criminally responsible at the age of ten (UNICEF, 2005). At thirteen an individual may take a part-time job but will not receive a statutory minimum wage until they finish compulsory education (Connexions, 2004; DTI, 2005). An individual can marry when they are sixteen (with parental consent) but they cannot vote in elections or buy an alcoholic drink in a bar until they are eighteen (Connexions, 2004). There are numerous examples which illustrate this point. Furthermore, policies such as the Government Green Paper *Every Child Matters* fail to acknowledge the experiences and potential service needs of young teenagers often classifying children as 'under 16' or '5–16'. Indeed, teenagers are only explicitly referred to in relation to teenage pregnancy (Weller, 2006b).

Part of the problem relating to inconsistency of definition is that the term 'children' represents both the age-based, biological status of a person as well as a relation between a parent and a child (Weller, 2006b). An adult is often referred to as someone's child whether they are 25 or 55 and 'offspring' is rarely an acceptable alternative (Weller, 2006b). Whilst it is likely that within certain contexts, particularly based around the family, some degree of interchangeability remains probable; it is nevertheless timely to pursue deconstructionist reading. Drawing on the work of authors such as Cixous important lessons can be learnt from deconstructing language and categories (Shurmer-Smith, 2000). In doing so, researchers will be more able to offer alternative concepts to the categories of 'child' or 'adult' and thus recognize that teenagers' experiences are liminal and are positioned on a boundary or threshold. I believe it is constructive to draw upon and adapt the notion of 'betweenness' outlined by Tooke (2000), who uses 'betweenness' to describe the positioning of research in a world between the researcher and the participant. Within the context of research with teenagers 'betweenness' refers to the positioning particularly of *young* teenagers (aged 13–16) as inhabiting a world distinct from both childhood and adulthood (Weller, 2006b).

Whilst acknowledging that teenagers are not an homogenous group, there are a number of common contexts which affect the lives of the majority to some degree. These factors are often regulated and influenced by systems which differ from those affecting children and young people (Weller, 2006b). Within the context of education policy, for example, the lives of young teenagers are shaped by the considerable amount of time that they spend in compulsory secondary schooling, working for exams, training to be 'citizens' and planning for their futures. Furthermore, the past two decades have witnessed a period of demonization and negative imagery, where teenagers are commonly represented as 'at-risk', 'in trouble' or 'in need' (Davies and Marken, 2000; Pain, 2003). A simple internet search or browse through contemporary newspaper archives reveals a myriad of issues, such as drug abuse, binge drinking, teenage pregnancy, anti-social behaviour and so on, all of which are obviously negative and portrayed as serious concerns for society (Weller, 2006b). A further key context which ultimately shapes teenagers' lived experiences is their representation and exclusion from public space (see Valentine, 2004). In particular recent policy moves in the UK ultimately criminalize their presence in such arenas. For example, an Anti-Social Behaviour Order (ASBO) can be placed upon anyone over the age of ten restricting where they are permitted to travel (Pain, 2003). Such derogatory representations shape the lives of many teenagers by presenting their actions and presence in public space as threatening and 'out-of-place'. In the media the 'troubled teenager' is a persistent theme (Bunting, 2004). Many youth organizations have been developed in order to monitor and control teenagers, especially those who are seen to be 'growing up' along less conventional trajectories (Wyn and White, 1997). Furthermore, few supportive services exist for teenagers in many areas of the UK (Millar, 2004). As a consequence many teenagers feel marginalized and left out of their communities, primarily because of their embodiment as young. The representation of teenagers as threatening is one of the major contexts influencing their lives, and is an arena which is often neglected if they are classified as children. This is particularly significant to the consideration of citizenship because age-based stereotypes can result in teenagers believing they are of lower status and have fewer rights (Wyn and White, 1997; Weller, 2003).

Researching teenagers' citizenship

The research project detailed in this book used a teenage-centred mixed methods approach comprising both quantitative and qualitative techniques over a period of eighteen months of fieldwork between 2000 and 2003. The study was based on the Isle of Wight (hereafter, the Island), a rural county located off the south coast of England. I spent the first eighteen years of my life living in a rural village on the Island, surrounded by thatched cottages, rolling hills and fields, woodlands and wild hedgerows. Some of my recollections fulfil the idyllic narratives of long summers, spatial freedoms and building dens associated with authors such as Enid Blyton. The hunt passed my house on Sunday mornings, and the village school and post office were significant places of news exchange and socialization. Whilst everything appeared idyllic, I outgrew my conscripted rose-tinted glasses well over a decade ago. Once jealous of the apparent freedom of the 'gangs' of kids that roamed freely, I saw a new disenfranchisement as a progressive cycle of locally labelled 'yobs' and 'no-hopers' lived out their popularly idealized childhood, not happily playing in the perpetual sunlight, but taking crack cocaine or heroin in the abandoned cottage three doors away from my house. Teenagers also reconditioned spaces in many positive ways, but many local decision-makers and other residents failed to recognize their contributions. I returned to my childhood haunts – both the area I grew up in and my former high school – in order to discover teenagers' current experiences.

Research locale

The Island is famed for its beautiful landscapes and picturesque villages, which receive 2.5 million visitors every year (Islandbreaks, 2003; see also Hollis, 1995). The teenagers who participated in my research reside in a wide range of places from tiny rural hamlets to seaside towns centred on tourism and more 'urban' council estates. Outwardly, the Island manifests a microcosm of all that is the quintessential English rural idyll – a safe haven for children to 'grow up' in. Nevertheless, whilst there are pockets of relative affluence, much of the Island is classified as a 'Rural Priority Area' suffering socio-economic problems and many areas suffer multiple disadvantage (Countryside Agency, 2000). Of the 48 electoral wards, 21 were ranked in the top 20 per cent of the most deprived areas in England when the study commenced (ONS, 2000). Two wards, home to some of the participants, were classified amongst the top 10 per cent of the most deprived areas in England (ONS, 2000). The *Isle of Wight Social Inclusion Strategy 2001–2005* offers several reasons for the high levels of deprivation. One key influence is the limited economic base centred upon seasonal tourism. The Island is one of the three counties in England with the lowest national average earnings (Countryside Agency, 2003a).

Whilst the research was undertaken within one research locale, this site may be described and interpreted into numerous differing micro-case studies, reflecting the diverse experiences of the participants involved. This research was not, therefore, essentialist in outlook and did not seek to make generalizations, but rather sought to gather rich information regarding teenagers' lived experiences of and engagement with citizenship.

The case study area was constructed on two levels: the 'community' level and the 'school' level. On the 'community' level, the Island provided the setting for the exploration of a myriad of teenagers' experiences of social exclusion, participation and citizenship. Whilst the study was carried out in a relatively deprived area, participants were not 'classified' as marginalized in other senses, for example, exclusion from school. With the exception of ethnicity[3] participants were from relatively mixed backgrounds.

The second level of the case study refers to the school in which the majority of participants were recruited and the locale for the analysis of citizenship education. This micro-level case study based in one co-educational, comprehensive school, 'Island High',[4] allowed a more in-depth exploration of teenagers' lived experiences of citizenship (Weller, 2006b). Teenagers attending the school are geographically dispersed, and travel from as far as the south and west coasts of the Island. Many of these areas are amongst the most economically deprived wards in the south-east of England. Nearly a quarter of teenagers at the school are entitled to free school meals compared to a 2001/2 national average of 15.3 per cent. In terms of academic achievement, the school falls below the national average of 56 per cent although it has seen a steady improvement in results since the mid 1990s. The school has been through a difficult and challenging period over the past decade.

Research methods

In all, around 600 participants contributed to the research via one or a number of mixed methods. At the 'community' level two key techniques, web-board discussions and a community radio phone-in (see Weller, 2006c), were utilized to ascertain broader views on teenagers' exclusion and participation. Techniques utilizing media such as the radio and internet developed out of a dynamic and evolving research process (Mason, 1996), which sought to home in on teenagers' own preferred communication techniques. A total of 50 participants including councillors, parents and teenagers contributed to radio and web-based discussions. These methods were coupled with observational work in citizenship lessons, teaching planning meetings and policy-orientated conferences.

At the 'school' level a number of techniques were used. Two surveys were administered to teenagers in the case study school. The first was completed by 425 teenagers (85 per cent response rate) across years 9, 10 and 11[5] and was administered prior to the introduction of compulsory citizenship education. The survey sought to explore teenagers' opinions on the new subject as well as to examine their exclusion from and participation in their local communities. A second, follow-up survey was then completed by 172 students (54 per cent response rate) in year 10 five months after the subject became compulsory. In this survey respondents were asked to comment on the value of the subject, both to their present and future lives. Subsequently, more in-depth work was carried out with a sub-sample of twenty teenagers in year 9. This year group was deemed by the school as the most able to accommodate in-depth involvement in a research project as they were yet to begin their GCSE studies.[6] Over a period of eighteen months the twenty teenagers, aged 13 and 14, worked on a number of in-depth methods including diary writing, photography and individual interviews/discussions in friendship groups, as well as informal chats and e-mail exchange. In their entirety, the research methods used were chosen and created to respond to different aspects of the research enquiry.

Involving teenagers

Whilst the ethical and methodological issues inherent in children-centred research reflect many of those apparent in the wider social sciences, the unique position that children and teenagers hold within society creates further issues for consideration (see, for example, Morrow and Richards, 1996; Mahon *et al.*, 1996; Mauthner, 1997; Holmes, 1998; Greig and Taylor, 1999; Lindsay, 2000). The construction of childhood as a period of innocence and dependency calls for research which is sensitive to the consideration of power (Matthews, 2001). More detailed explorations of the ethical and methodological issues that arose during the course of my research can be found in Barker and Weller (2003a; 2003b) and Weller (2004b; 2006c).

In order to go some way to counter the power imbalances between myself and participants, teenagers were actively included in the research process through two practices of negotiation. In the first practice, two research consultants, my stepchildren (then aged 13 and 16), provided advice on the structure, layout, content and wording of information sheets and the implementation of each method, in addition to offering general research ideas and approaches. During the second set of negotiations I worked directly with participants in the case study area, through pre-pilot trials of each technique. This second consultation approach encompassed a larger and more diverse group of respondents, which enabled each technique to be evaluated more thoroughly. Whilst this two-stranded consultation approach did not satisfy the idealistic notion of providing participants with the opportunity to define the research agenda, it did make important steps towards a more realistic compromise (see also Barker and Weller, 2003b). Participants chose their own pseudonyms which are used throughout this book.

The structure of the book

The final section of this introductory chapter outlines the structure of the book. Chapter 2 is concerned with teenagers' problematic relationship with dominant understandings of citizenship. I examine debates around the contested notion of young teenagers as citizens by providing an in-depth theoretical exploration of teenagers' status in society as future citizens and their role within democracy and local and national democratic arenas. I will also explore constructions of young teenagers as incompetent, incomplete and apathetic. Finally I introduce some more recent perspectives which have begun to include children and young teenagers, both theoretically and practically, for example, the 'New Feminist Perspectives on Citizenship' and the 'New Social Studies of Childhood' and I discuss the implications these have upon teenagers' citizenship and citizenship education.

Chapter 3 looks at the introduction of citizenship education in England as an illustration of what happens when citizenship moves into schools. From September 2002, citizenship education became compulsory for children and teenagers in secondary education in England. This new wave of teaching democracy is seen as a distinct shift from the civics education of the 1960s and 1970s to that based upon discussion and participation. Importantly, I examine the specifics of citizenship education as a policy and question whether involving children will raise new issues beyond the government's current agenda. This chapter is concerned with pedagogy and I will discuss the nature of the curriculum, how it was developed and how contemporary citizenship education differs from past teachings. Importantly, this chapter will explore young teenagers' own views on the implementation of the citizenship curriculum.

Continuing with the theme of citizenship in school, chapter 4 explores teenagers' experiences of participation in decision-making. I not only draw attention to the importance of the resources and spaces provided for active citizenship, such as school councils, but also examine the significance of relationships with teaching staff. For example, when deficit models of childhood and citizenship are disregarded in the classroom, this has a positive impact upon engagement with the subject. When teenagers feel that they are treated like adults or perhaps as equals, and where they are afforded the opportunity actively to make decisions over their learning, they are more likely to be engaged in citizenship education.

Chapter 5 examines teenagers' own practices and experiences of citizenship. Using several case studies I highlight examples of young teenagers who have devised creative and resourceful ways in which to redefine and reconstruct everyday spaces and identities. Examining young teenagers' own definitions challenges conventional understandings of community and identity, which are implicit facets of citizenship. Many of these identifications are with more lifestyle-based communities of practice. These examples include developing skate-park facilities, campaigning for the preservation of youth centres and carving out spaces in marginalized areas of their environments, thus highlighting alternative modes of civic engagement and social capital.

Chapter 6 explores teenagers' encounters of inclusion within and exclusion from local governance by exploring the extent to which participants felt listened to by local decision-makers. Initially, I examine teenagers' experiences of participation in decision-making in the community with particular reference to youth parliaments and forums. Subsequently, I will argue that, whilst positive attempts have been made to increase the opportunity for involvement by young people, local decision-makers have used limited methods of gathering opinions and have made uninformed decisions on behalf of teenagers without thorough consultation. Whilst such moves are a step in the right direction, they need to be made *with* teenagers and not *for* teenagers in order to curb growing resentment.

The final chapter will synthesize and analyse the main themes explored in the previous chapters. I will argue for a new approach to citizenship which upgrades the status of teenagers, particularly within the classroom. I call for a cumulative notion of citizenship where children, teenagers and adults alike are all represented as full citizens who learn, develop and exert different forms of citizenship in different arenas at different stages in their lives. This concluding chapter aims to shift the direction of citizenship education discourse and dominant societal understandings of citizenship towards recognizing that teenagers exert their own practices of citizenship when citizenship is viewed through a more cosmopolitan lens. The chapter will also consider the resonance of this work for contexts beyond England.

Chapter 2

Young teenagers' relationship with citizenship

Introducing citizenship

Those active in the children-led anti-war demonstrations in 2003 were not praised for their political engagement. Instead they were patronized and punished for their involvement. One girl protested against the thirty-day exclusion imposed by her school, taking it to the High Court. Despite winning her case the judge deemed her to be a 'very silly girl' (SchNEWS, 2004), alluding to the idea that she did not really know what she was doing. Indeed, dominant accounts suggested that many of the children and young people were not competent enough to understand either the issues or their actions, despite evidence to suggest that their justifications for participating in the protests were well thought through and certainly not simply a way of avoiding going to school (Cunningham and Lavalette, 2004). The children-led anti-war protests are a compelling example of the way in which young people *do* participate in acts of citizenship. The responses of the authorities towards such actions also provide a powerful example of young people's problematic relationship with citizenship as it is constructed within contemporary British society. Within a climate of fear regarding the political apathy of the young this is, indeed, paradoxical. It is the purpose of this book to highlight further examples of this contradiction and to explore young teenagers' problematic relationship with dominant constructions of 'citizenship'.

With concerns about the renewal of civil society, citizenship has come to the fore in contemporary Britain and has become a popular buzzword imbued with political meaning (Cockburn, 1998; Crace, 2000; Marston and Mitchell, 2004; Jochum *et al.*, 2005). As Lister *et al.* argue:

'Vocabularies of citizenship' and their meanings vary according to social, political and cultural context and reflect different historical legacies.

(2003: 235)

Since the 1980s renewed emphasis on citizenship has been in part due to factors which have challenged the centrality of the state, such as the growing significance of the European Union (EU), globalization, the quest for regional autonomy in some areas, as well as international migration (Lister, 1998). Currently, citizenship is most commonly used in policy and media debates around both immigration and youth-centred policies for it is these groups that often challenge the notion of national citizenship (Gifford, 2004). New migrants to Britain are now expected to pass a test and attend a citizenship ceremony in order to acquire a passport and British citizenship; a feat which would undoubtedly challenge many of those already considered as British citizens (Bhattacharyya, 2004; Harkin, 2005; Travis, 2005). Citizenship is, therefore, primarily used in debates about 'who belongs?'. For policy-makers this raises many concerns about how to train individuals to be responsible (British) citizens.

The consideration of citizenship is inherently tied to understandings of democracy. Quintessentially, democracy may be defined as collective decision-making and it is a form of governance that is almost universally advocated (Beetham and Boyle, 1998; Barnett and Low, 2004). In contemporary society, democracy is a dynamic concept, often culturally specific following differing ideological paths (see Giddens, 2000a). Akin to democracy, citizenship as a concept has many competing definitions, although the liberal perspective is arguably the most dominant in Western society. Citizenship may be defined using a number of terms including legal, philosophical and/or socio-political (Faulks, 1998). Whilst such competing understandings exist, citizenship is nevertheless a popular concept amongst a wide range of groups from differing political persuasions (Lister, 1998; Faulks, 2000). As a concept it has been important both in New Right thinking as well as in New Labour's 'left' perspective (Lister, 1998). These disparate perspectives do share an understanding of citizenship as consisting of a number of common dimensions, such as 'rights', 'obligations/duties' and a relationship with the state/political institutions. As Faulks summarizes:

> citizenship is a membership status, which contains a package of rights, duties and obligations, and which implies equality, justice and autonomy.
>
> (2000: 13)

Rights and duties form the basis of many perspectives on citizenship, although different schools of thought place different degrees of emphasis upon each. Originating from Roman jurisprudence, Audi (1996) suggests a 'right' is an advantageous position afforded to an individual by the moral code of a society. A right may be either positive, for example the right to free speech, or negative, for instance immunity from torture. A right may be either active or passive, for example, the former might include the right to self-defence (Audi, 1996). A right may be either moral or legal (Flew, 2000).

A right may also be absolute, in that it applies whatever the consequences, or it may be prima facie, only applying if the consequences are not greater than the right itself (Audi, 1996). It is likely that the rights of one person may conflict with those of another (Osler and Starkey, 2005b). Furthermore, rights are inherently bound to status; for example, civil rights are those afforded to citizens, and children's rights are those afforded to children. Human rights are problematic in definition, encompassing civil, economic, political, cultural and social aspects (Taylor, 2000). They are frequently perceived to be synonymous with natural rights or entitlements received at birth, and are used to provide a universal standard by which societies are monitored (Audi, 1996; Baggini, 2002). John Locke, in his 'social contract theory', wrote of the natural rights of citizens to 'life, liberty and property' (Heywood, 1992). The concept of natural rights is highly contested and many view the existence of rights as socially constructed (Baggini, 2002). In citizenship discourse the notion of 'rights' is often seen to infer a relationship with 'duties' or 'responsibilities' (Audi, 1996). Duties may be active, for example participating in the local community, or they may be defined in more passive terms such as paying taxes. The way different writers have expressed elements such as 'rights' and 'duties', or indeed the focus that is placed on each, varies between different schools of thought. For example, liberal approaches tend to focus more on 'rights', whilst communitarian thought centres upon 'duties'. Even amongst feminist thought views differ on the emphasis placed on both rights and duties (see, for example, Lister, 1997a; 1997b).

There has been a long-standing connection between geography and citizenship although the consideration of citizenship has often been implicit within geographical studies (Painter and Philo, 1995). Geographical research on citizenship has principally been concerned with themes such as migration, belonging and access to resources. In particular, emphasis has been placed upon the impact of globalization on citizenship bound to the nation-state. Geographers have also been concerned with electoral politics and participation. Barnett and Low argue that geographers' focus on the construction of bounded territories has resulted in a reluctance to engage with space at the level of the nation-state. Instead, dominant lines of thought in geography centre upon spaces as:

> uneven, relational, reticulated, blurry, stratified, folded over, porous and so on.
>
> (2004: 9)

At the same time geography offers new ways of considering more alternative spaces of citizenship and democracy. Such spaces are numerous and eclectic ranging from the nation-state to more micro-spaces, and from more conventional to alternative arenas. Staeheli and Mitchell (2004) argue that such spaces are important in moulding the political actions that occur within them. As highlighted in chapter 1, this book assumes a geographical analysis of teenagers' citizenship, arguing that it is by exploring the spatial that examples and understandings of teenagers' citizenship become apparent. Space(s) and place(s) inherently shape rights, duties and a sense of belonging (Painter and Philo, 1995). Here, particular emphasis will be placed upon micro-spaces or places of the everyday experience.

In order to frame the discussions about learning and practising citizenship in chapters 4, 5 and 6, this chapter engages with complex debates surrounding teenagers' problematic relationship with citizenship and, in particular, their societal status as citizens of the future. The chapter begins by exploring two dominant but conflicting understandings of citizenship. Subsequently, it highlights the ways in which key writers on citizenship have neglected the young, constructing them as incompetent, incomplete and apathetic. Finally, attention will turn to more contemporary understandings of citizenship which argue for a more inclusive and flexible approach that acknowledges the different dimensions in which an individual or collective may be regarded as, or seen to be acting as, a citizen.

Contested understandings of citizenship

Over time the concept of citizenship has developed through a number of phases to produce differing ideas and understandings (Faulks, 2000). Above I have provided a brief exploration of two influential and dominant areas of thought, beginning with civic republicanism and the communitarian approach and followed by the liberal perspective. These schools of thought provide the foundation for what is considered to be more conventional understandings of citizenship and I look at them in more detail now.

The influence of civic republicanism and the communitarian approach

The origins of citizenship theory can be traced back to the works of Aristotle and the city-states of ancient Greece (Crick, 2000; Faulks, 2000; Dwyer, 2004; Leighton, 2004). This civic republican vision of citizenship focused upon obligations and civic virtue, and as Faulks highlights:

> from birth, citizens internalised the values of active citizenship, greatly influencing the content and depth of its practice.
>
> (2000: 16)

The civic republican perspective promotes citizenship as a practice upholding the notion of *active* citizenship (Lister, 1998). This approach makes a key distinction between the public and private spheres. In these terms there is minimal state intervention in the private sphere and some regulation in the public sphere to maintain order between different groups within society (Osler and Starkey, 2005b).

Citizenship in ancient Greece focused around the polis, a much smaller space than the modern nation-state, with 'the many' or 'the poor' in rule (Heywood, 1992), although the system was inherently exclusive as it only extended to *male* citizens (it did also omit some groups of men including slaves). (Male) citizens were actively involved in the polis through meetings and referendums, and held a position in government at some point in their lives through a rota system (Heywood, 1992).

Civic republicanism was also influential during the Roman Empire until the empire grew too large to sustain a notion of citizenship based around kinship in small close-knit communities. Elements of civic republicanism remained significant in the eighteenth century, for example, Machiavelli's notion of city-states. Nevertheless, this approach declined in popularity with the onset of a more dominant liberal perspective in the late seventeenth century. Key elements underpinning civic republicanism have, however, been influential in the development of more contemporary communitarian perspectives on citizenship (Dwyer, 2004).

In general, the communitarian notion of citizenship denounces individualism, instead focusing on obligations and the sharing of norms and values for the common good of the community (Lawson, 2001; Dwyer, 2004; Gifford, 2004). Unlike liberalism, citizenship from a communitarian perspective focuses on solidarity in collectives and participation in the community, holding moral standings at a communal level rather than the individual (Brown, 1997; Osler and Starkey, 2005b). This approach also recognizes the influence of social context and/or community upon individuals (Dwyer, 2004; Jochum *et al.*, 2005). The communitarian perspective, therefore, focuses upon obligations over individual rights. As Dwyer highlights:

> The communitarian goal is to encourage participatory politics in which people recognize their social obligations as well as their individual rights. This they actively achieve within specific communities.
>
> (2004: 28)

Communitarian understandings of citizenship take on a number of different forms from 'conservative communitarianism' which accepts inequality and hierarchy, to 'radical communitarianism' which calls for the abolition of an hierarchical notion of the common good. Whilst communitarianism generally functions at the more local level, some authors have envisaged communitarianism at the level of the state. Communitarian perspectives have been subject to criticism, and in particular the focus on community raises many questions relating to the inclusion and exclusion of individuals from different communities (Dwyer, 2004).

Liberal perspectives

In essence the liberal perspective upholds citizenship as a right and as a status (Lister, 1997a; 1998; Jochum *et al.*, 2005). The liberal approach to citizenship focuses upon individual rights, with the individual in pursuit of her/his idea of 'the good', as Brown highlights:

> politics are defined as actions the individual takes to get the things s/he wants from the state or other citizens, while mitigating the state's interference in this pursuit of happiness.
>
> (1997: 6)

Whilst some emphasis is placed upon duties in order to maintain society and allocate resources (Faulks, 2000) rights are the key focus of the liberal perspective. In these terms the state plays only a minimal role in the lives of individuals focusing primarily on promoting rights (Dwyer, 2004). Unlike the communitarian approach sparse emphasis is placed upon considerations of community.

As Faulks (2000) suggests, contemporary understandings of citizenship are bound to the emergence of the liberal state, the roots of which date back to the late sixteenth century. A number of societal changes were significant in the development of the early liberal thought on citizenship, for example, the pronouncement of state boundaries in the eighteenth century, the growth of consensual government and the separation of religion from politics to create secular states, thus challenging rule by monarchy (Painter and Philo, 1995; Faulks, 2000; Dwyer, 2004). Remonstrations such as the political revolutions in America in 1776 and in particular in France in 1789 were significant in the creation of modernity as the population replaced the monarch as sovereign (Faulks, 2000; Heywood, 1992). Such transformations led to citizen identities which were tied to a bounded region: the modern nation-state (Painter and Philo, 1995). Early liberal thought on the rights of the individual, therefore, came about at the same time as the emergence of the parliamentary state in Britain (Marston and Mitchell, 2004). Modern thought on citizenship stemmed from the works of early liberal philosophers, such as John Locke and later John Stuart Mill, many of whom argued that the promotion of civil and political rights would secure the freedom of the individual from heavy state rule (Faulks, 2000; Dwyer, 2004). Thomas Hobbes, for example, was influential in highlighting connections between citizenship and egalitarianism (Faulks, 2000). Many of these early writers also believed that citizens needed both 'factual knowledge', as well as experience in order to participate in democracy (Tooley, 2000).

As Faulks (2000) describes, historically the development of citizenship may be likened to 'expanding circles' gradually becoming more inclusive and incorporating different sections of society. Nineteenth-century Britain witnessed many campaigns for a more inclusive franchise, and by 1884 (Reform Act) there was a universal vote for men, with women's suffrage in 1928 (Equal Franchise Act) (Heywood, 1992). This form of democracy embraced a representative approach whereby 'the many' took part in regular elections to select a candidate who they believed best able to fulfil their political, social, economic and cultural needs and desires. Despite this, democracy in the nineteenth century was not always viewed favourably for fear that a broad franchise would prove a threat to a (wealthy) person's liberty (Heywood, 1992). Nevertheless, a new inclusive status emerged for the citizen:

> Thus the history of modern citizenship can in part be understood as a series of bargains and trade offs, whereby elites seek to maintain their power through managing the effects of social change and containing the demands of social movements through concessions in the form of rights.
>
> (Faulks, 2000: 25)

Whilst Faulk's (2000) historical description of citizenship focuses on expanding circles, citizenship can also contract reducing citizenship rights to different groups. Furthermore, the extent to which 'the many' have equal access to power remains questionable in twenty-first-century Britain. Whilst representative democracy does prevent stagnation as politicians can be replaced regularly, 'the many' still equates to the adult population, and those elected to represent 'the many' are disproportionately middle-class, white and male (Heywood, 1992; Beetham and Boyle, 1998).

Akin to liberalism more generally there is not one universal liberal theory of citizenship but a range of understandings all of which hold central the notion of individualism (Barnett and Low, 2004; Dwyer, 2004). 'Libertarian liberals', for example, believe in the market as the appropriate mechanism for the distribution of goods, and argue for laissez-faire governance with the state intervening only in order to maintain basic civil and political rights. Alternatively the 'egalitarian liberal' stance argues that the market does not necessarily distribute goods justly and, therefore, upholds the need for some state intervention to ensure social rights and the freedom of the individual (Dwyer, 2004). One such egalitarian liberal thinker was T.H. Marshall. Marshall's eminent work synthesized liberal and social democratic perspectives, defining a nation-state-based citizenship as:

> a status bestowed on those who are full members of a community. All who possess the status are equal with respect to rights and duties with which the status is endowed.
>
> (1950: 28–29)

Writing just after the end of the Second World War, Marshall viewed citizenship as a status, where all citizens are equal even if other inequalities persist. Whilst Marshall did place some emphasis on the importance of duties such as paying taxes and participating in compulsory education and work (Dwyer, 2004), his key contribution focused on a model of citizenship consisting of three rights-based elements: civil citizenship or freedom of speech and thought; political citizenship or the right to participate; and social citizenship or the right to welfare (Marston and Mitchell, 2004). Within Britain the three aspects of citizenship were seen by Marshall to have developed historically over three centuries, commencing with the evolution of civil citizenship brought about by the decline in feudalism and the growth of capitalism, for example, the Poor Laws between the fifteenth and seventeenth centuries (Dwyer, 2004). Subsequently, the nineteenth-century extension of the franchise bore political citizenship. Social citizenship was not seen to have arisen until the emergence of, for example, twentieth-century trade unionism (Isin and Wood, 1999). In particular, Marshall focused on the significance of social rights through the growth of the welfare state in dealing with inequalities (France, 1998). Whilst Marshall's work has received some criticism, for example for placing too much emphasis on the nation-state (see Dwyer, 2004 for a summary), there are a number of important aspects which continue to be influential. First, the three elements Marshall puts forward – civil, political and social rights – provide an important basis for examining exclusion from full citizenship (Dwyer, 2004). Second, Marshall's conceptualization remains valuable because it provides useful insights into the changing relationship between citizenship and capitalism (Marston and Mitchell, 2004; Biesta and Lawy, 2006). Third, Marshall's construction of citizenship has played a significant role in the formulation of contemporary citizenship education. Finally, the more recent growth of neo-liberal perspectives signals a return to early concerns about state intervention (Marston and Mitchell, 2004).

More generally, liberal perspectives on citizenship have received some criticism. Faulks (2000) describes the liberal approach as 'thin' in that it is subject to market dominance and the power of elites. Furthermore, focus on the abstract individual has failed to acknowledge differences and inequalities within society that constrain access to rights and duties (Faulks, 2000). Osler and Starkey further this by suggesting:

> Liberal democracies are potentially fragile, in particular where apathy and fatalism allow strongly nationalist or xenophobic parties to gain political control, as happened notoriously in Germany in 1932–33.
>
> (2005b: 35)

Civic republican/communitarian and liberal perspectives place very different emphases on the purpose and definition of citizenship. In particular these alternative approaches focus upon different understandings of the role of the market, the nation-state and community, thus highlighting different perspectives on space. Moreover, these stances also place different emphases upon the importance of rights and duties, as well as the role of the individual within different contexts.

During the 1980s and early 1990s the then Conservative Government in Britain advocated an individualistic liberal notion of 'active' citizenship (France, 1998; Jochum et al., 2005) which authors such as Biesta and Lawy (2006) have described as a privatized notion of citizenship. Since the 1980s there has been a distinct shift in formal British politics from a notion of citizenship based upon 'rights' to that based on 'duties' with, for example, the introduction of the Child Support Act 1993 by the then Conservative Government (Lister, 1998). The New Labour Government has perpetuated this move by advocating a citizenship based upon obligations, promoting in particular the notion that social rights have to be earned (Lister, 1998; Lawson, 2001; Dwyer, 2004; Jochum et al., 2005). In these terms the current New Labour Government is positioned nearer to the communitarian perspective on citizenship than the liberal (Dwyer, 2004).

Young teenagers' problematic relationship with citizenship

It is not uncommon for discussions on the conceptualization of citizenship to exclude children and young teenagers. Indeed, it is often only within the context of education policy and some aspects of welfare policy that a relationship between teenagers and citizenship is acknowledged. The transition to adulthood is, however, an important time for teenagers' citizenship as Lister et al. state:

> More than at other points of the life-course, youth is a time when the relationship to citizenship is in a state of flux.
>
> (2003: 236)

Conceptually, citizenship presents the foundations for full participation in a community (Johnston et al., 2000) and as I now discuss for children and young teenagers this is somewhat problematic.

Citizenship and competency

Children and young teenagers' problematic relationship with dominant conceptualizations of citizenship undeniably relates to issues of competency. Past work in psychology, for example, has principally focused on children's lack of competency (Marchant and Kirby, 2004). More widely children are regarded as vulnerable and incomplete (Pilcher, 1995), whereby decisions are made by adults in the 'best interests' of the 'incompetent child' (Gittens, 1998). Although this is commonly held as an integral part of parental responsibility it may also, as Gittens (1998) suggests, reinforce ideas of 'the child' as private property. Children and young teenagers are, therefore, regarded as incompetent and in need of training in the ways of contemporary citizenship. Indeed, Marshall (1965) professed that children were not developed enough to be trusted; a point reinforced in Kantian ethics. Kant regarded the differential treatment of children from adults as valid (Schapiro, 1999), and referred to children as 'passive citizens'; the significance of this term will be revisited in subsequent chapters. Plato, Aristotle and Freud also believed that childhood ceased when reason became apparent (Kennedy, 2000). An increase in the ability to reason, therefore, allowed heightened autonomy in Kantian terms. Many key authors and schools of thought have, therefore, commonly regarded children and teenagers as citizens-in-the-making.

What is, however, particularly problematic is the identification of competency with biological age (Valentine, 2000), thus creating a false dichotomy between adulthood and childhood. For as Neale notes:

> There is an underlying assumption that it is only when (or if) young people can accommodate to the world of adulthood that they will have something worth saying and can be taken seriously. In other words, their inclusion is conditional on their assuming 'adult' modes of behaving and communicating.
>
> (2004: 15)

The notion that young people are citizens-in-the-making, in need of training in the ways of citizenship, is only validated by the societal acceptance that childhood can be demarcated, sectioned off and excluded from several key aspects of citizenship. The notion of democracy has received opposition from those who regard 'the many' as too ignorant or uneducated (Beetham and Boyle, 1998), and yet justifiably there would be outrage if the adult population had to prove competency in order to, for example, exercise their right to vote. Whilst it is important to acknowledge that there are recognizable differences between the thought-processes of toddlers and young teenagers (Neale, 2004), the rigid definitions of childhood associated with developmental stages, the end of which is demarcated by the age of eighteen in the UK, is problematic and brings into question legislation which delineates the end of childhood to a specific age. Problematically, this boundary also signifies the acquisition of full citizenship (Hall *et al.*, 1999).

In contrast Valentine (2004) views competence as a performative concept rather than related to biology. This argument is reinforced by numerous instances where children and young teenagers demonstrate their role in society as competent social and political actors, for example

as carers for their parents or as child soldiers. It is a very Western conceptualization of childhood that upholds the dependency thesis. Indeed, there
are many arenas in which children and young people may exhibit greater
competency than adults. One example of this is the role many children in
Europe and the USA play in peer support schemes, mediation, conflict resolution and counselling in both primary and secondary schools. Wyness
(2000) argues that children are much more likely to understand peer
group interaction in the playground and are also likely to be more
approachable than teaching staff. Within this context children may be
regarded as more competent than adults. In some arenas discourse has
shifted focus away from age-based competency to that centred on individual abilities and greater recognition of children and teenagers'
responsibilities. Arguably such moves have the potential to enhance
young people's status in society (Mayall, 2002). For example, the NSSC,
outlined in chapter 1, have to some degree changed views of children and
young people's competency in both research and policy arenas.
Nevertheless, there remains a wider societal reluctance to view children
and young people in this way (Marchant and Kirby, 2004).

Citizens-in-the-making

Children and young teenagers are also portrayed as incomplete. Marshall's
(1950) influential work on citizenship constructed young people as 'citizens-
in-the-making' affording them few rights (James and James, 2004). This
understanding of children and young teenagers' relationship with citizenship dominates legislation and policy within Britain. As chapter 3 will
highlight, the purpose of contemporary citizenship education is centred
upon creating 'future responsible citizens'. A number of factors have
fuelled this view of young people's citizenship status. The modern conceptualization of childhood and the placing of children into the private
domain coupled with the common notion of 'citizen' as synonymous with
'worker' fosters the kinds of challenges faced by the young anti-war pro-
testors in 2003. Moreover, the marginalization of children and young
teenagers is bound to the constitutional exclusion from full citizenship for
those under the age of eighteen in Britain (Roche, 1999). Children and
young teenagers are, therefore, rarely regarded as 'political' by virtue of
their exclusion from the political elements of citizenship. According to
James and James (2004) it is legislation which is significant in positioning
children within society. As chapter 1 highlighted, within the UK both legislation and policy follow a very fluid notion of the progression to
adulthood, although since the Family Law Reform Act 1969 the age of
eighteen has come to represent the start of adulthood. It is this artificial
boundary that marks out children as non- or incomplete citizens. This
demarcation may be further reinforced with the introduction of citizenship

ceremonies for 18-year-olds. Such 'celebrations' are intended to mark the transition to adulthood, to promote a sense of Britishness and to encourage engagement in formal politics.

Within late-modernity, Cockburn (2000) suggests, children's autonomy and citizenship has been eroded. Focusing on the seventeenth- and eighteenth-century clearance of street children, reformists removed children's level of agency by placing them in the private domain, thus separating the life-worlds of children and adults. Until then children had been viewed as their parents' property; as workers in, for example, the factories of the Industrial Revolution. Paradoxically, it was the development of children's rights to welfare that removed the level of citizenship they had been previously afforded (James and James, 2004). The equation between citizen and worker remains prevalent, for example the EU defines 'citizen as worker' (Euronet, 2000; Lister *et al.*, 2003). The equation between work and citizenship was also reinforced by young people (aged 16–23) in Lister *et al.*'s study, many of whom argued that the unemployed were often considered to be second-class citizens. Such portrayals have implications for those under the age of eighteen as the dominant Western conceptualization of childhood denies children access to full-time paid work (Roche, 1999). In many spheres, including the EU, there are no formal mechanisms for young people's citizenship in these terms (Euronet, 2000). Children and young teenagers are, therefore, constructed out of society and denied personhood (Ennew, 1994).

Legislation and policy specifically relating to education has also played an important role in constructing childhood. Nineteenth-century education reforms were arguably a response to the emergence of a perceived connection between delinquency and youth (Hendrick, 1997; James and James, 2004). The placing of children into schools and the construction of a particular type of common 'national child' rendered education policy, in part, a form of social control. A universal view of childhood also exists in policy today with the underlying assumption that children need to be taught about and to learn how to be effective members of society, as well as, 'proper children' (James and James, 2004: 123). Children and young people are, therefore, by association excluded from many elements of political and social life. The policy quest for a regulated, universal 'national childhood' is at odds with the seemingly positive steps towards encouraging active participation outlined in the citizenship curriculum (James and James, 2004). Young people, therefore, became citizens-in-the-making through compulsory education and as a result were denied access to the spaces of modern citizenship (Cockburn, 2000). It was in the twentieth century that new understandings of childhood emerged, and whilst separated from the adult domain, children came to be regarded as people (rather than property) who in the twenty-first century were afforded rights (Osler and Starkey, 2005a). It is in the development of children's rights that a new space for young people's citizenship may emerge.

The paradox of teenage apathy

In the 1990s Harry Enfield, a contemporary British comedian, created a character which he used in television sketch shows (see Enfield, 1997). In his first appearance, the character, Kevin, has his thirteenth birthday. As the clock strikes midnight Kevin transforms from a sweet, well-behaved child to a stroppy and rude teenager. This representation of teenagers has resonated throughout the media. More recently, comedian Catherine Tate's argumentative teenage character, Lauren, has become famous for her catchphrase 'Am I bovvered?!' (BBC, 2006). Whilst these are arguably light-hearted representations they do illustrate the dominant way in which teenagers are portrayed. Again, this understanding presents a paradox. Children and young teenagers are on the one hand regarded as incompetent and incomplete, and yet on the other hand, young teenagers in particular are frequently viewed as apathetic and so by definition are making an active decision not to be 'bovvered'. At the same time the actions of many young people are also simultaneously portrayed as threatening particularly in public space (Valentine, 2004; Osler and Starkey, 2005b). These conflicting representations of teenagers do much to shape the way in which teenagers are seen by the wider community.

Concerns about young people's disengagement are often derived from statistical measures such as voter turnout at elections. Those aged 18 to 24 were amongst the least likely to vote in both the 2001 and 2005 General Elections (CYPU, 2002; ESRC, 2005). Indeed, not only were the youngest quartile of the franchise least likely to vote, but turnout has been in sharp decline in the UK amongst this group over the past 100 years echoing trends in other parts of Europe (Jowell and Park, 1998; CYPU, 2002). Whilst those younger than eighteen are implicitly excluded from such measures, they are nevertheless also often regarded as apathetic. Two foundations for teenage apathy are outlined by the Children and Young People's Unit (CYPU, 2002; see also ESRC, 2005). The first suggests that the level of political engagement is dependent on an individual's stage in the life-course. In this scenario, voters are less likely to be apathetic when they have a stake in society as, for example, taxpayers (CYPU, 2002). Such a proposal verifies the idea that disengagement relates to a lack of place or stake in society. The second foundation for teenage apathy relates to the idea that the current generation of young people is different from past generations, in some way inherently more apathetic than their predecessors, and that such apathy will not change with stage in the life-course (CYPU, 2002). Putnam's (2000) influential work on social capital describes what he perceives to be changes in civic engagement in the USA. Putnam (2000) also upholds the notion of generational difference in civic engagement suggesting a general decline. Indeed, it is apparent that generations experience different economic, political and social changes within their societies, and it is perhaps because of such global, national and even local transformations that what is meant by 'political' also needs to be challenged. Cross-generational comparisons are, therefore, problematic.

In 2002 the CYPU looked more closely at political apathy with 60 participants aged 14–19 (CYPU, 2002). Politicians were frequently perceived by participants as white, wealthy, patronising, older men. Many felt that not only did politicians engage solely with people who were old enough to vote, but that political rhetoric, especially broadcast through the media, focused only upon the negative aspects of youth and the actions of a minority, including issues such as drug abuse (CYPU, 2002). Furthermore, there was a general lack of understanding regarding the function and workings of political institutions. Although the CYPU did acknowledge that many young people engage in alternative forms of political activity, these were referred to as 'non-traditional' and included petitioning, campaigning and protest, often at the local level. Historically, those who are marginalized within society find that such actions are their only successful means of participation. Local action is often a response to the manifestations of national policies within individual communities (CYPU, 2002). As a result of the consultation, a 'young person's agenda for democracy' was formulated, which outlined the need for politicians to take on board, without assumptions or prejudices, the opinions of those not yet old enough to vote; to communicate using accessible language; and to respect that young people are not an homogenous group (CYPU, 2002). Recommendations for the government included: providing information, particularly through citizenship education; and increasing the franchise by lowering the age of voting (CYPU, 2002). The consultation also highlighted areas in which the ever-influential media could contribute to political engagement using, for example, television programmes, such as soap operas, to raise important issues.

Dominant representations of teenagers as apathetic are problematic. Common measures such as low voter turnout fail to include those under the age of eighteen, as well as presenting a very rigid definition of politics and political action. Participants in Lister et al.'s (2001) study suggested that it was more responsible not to vote than to 'just tick anything'. Roker et al. (1999) also cite a number of cases where there has been a marked increase in young people joining and participating in social/political groups. Arguably, many young people now engage in areas such as the politics of consumerism (Stuart, 2000; Valentine, 2000). The subsequent chapters of this book will highlight numerous ways in which many young teenagers actively engage in their local communities and schools.

Despite young teenagers' problematic relationship with dominant understandings of citizenship several authors, drawing upon the NSSC, have utilized a more social definition of citizenship. Neale (2004) in her work with young children has synthesized notions of children both as welfare dependents and as citizens to argue that citizenship should be a nurturing process where the young are afforded experiences through meaningful participation. Viewing young people in these terms acknowledges their competency and does indeed afford them with some citizenship status. Nevertheless, it is still important to recognize the power of more conventional and dominant understandings of citizenship in shaping the spaces and opportunities the young are afforded for active participation. It is useful to draw upon Kjørholt's (2004) work with the Norwegian 'Try Yourself' project which sought to provide funding for children's self-directed cultural activities. The scheme regarded children as *equal to* but *different from* adults in that the application process differed from adult procedures. Whilst this was a valid attempt at embracing difference amongst citizens, the differential treatment of children raises questions about the extent to which they are really viewed as equal.

The final section of this chapter builds upon the ideas of both authors such as Neale (2004), as well as writers on alternative understandings of citizenship in order to present a more fitting and meaningful conceptualization. It begins by briefly highlighting three alternative conceptualizations of citizenship, drawing upon post-modern/post-structural, cosmopolitan and feminist perspectives to offer a more inclusive notion of citizenship. Second, the children's rights movement and the growth in opportunities for young people's participation will be highlighted as more practical examples of the way in which citizenship can be reframed to include the actions and experiences of children and teenagers.

Conceptual moves towards inclusive citizenship

There are a number of contemporary conceptualizations of citizenship which have the potential to provide a more useful framework for teenagers' citizenship. This book will draw upon elements from all three of the following perspectives, in particular new feminist perspectives. These approaches are not mutually exclusive but intertwined, and in some cases complementary in their arguments.

Post-modern and post-structural insights

Post-structural political thought has made an important contribution to citizenship studies and has many implications for the re-examination of the human subject (Brown, 1997). Such thought has deconstructed conventional understandings of citizenship associated with liberalism and communitarianism. In particular, these reconstructions have rejected and critiqued the exclusive nature of the 'liberal citizen' and the static identity inherent within it (Brown, 1997). This is of importance in the consideration of children and teenagers' citizenship, as liberal politics has denied the influence of political citizenship within the home and family. Marshall's definition has also been criticized for placing too much emphasis upon rights and too little upon struggle (Isin and Wood, 1999). As Brown (1997) notes, whilst a post-structural theory of radical democracy takes on board notions relating to communitarianism, it also opposes the focus on a single societal moral code.

Many post-modern perspectives challenge the connection between citizenship and rigid national boundaries (Faulks, 2000), arguing for a more fluid definition. Drawing upon children's experiences, Skelton's (2005) description of the political identities of those living on the Caribbean island of Montserrat is a pertinent example of this complexity. Residents of this British overseas territory may be considered as British citizens or subjects, Montserratians or migrants from other countries/territories in the Caribbean, and many participate in and celebrate both aspects of the Commonwealth and the end of British slavery (Skelton, 2005). In line with such examples several authors have proposed the notion of 'multiple citizenship' (see, for example, Heater, 1990). This alternative perspective acknowledges that individuals feel allegiance to a multitude of political spheres and moves away from the idea of citizenship tied to the nation-state:

> what postmodern citizenship demands is that boundaries between political communities are not perpetually closed, either materially or culturally, and that many of the rights and responsibilities of citizenship extend beyond administrative boundaries.
>
> (Faulks, 2000: 168)

Many post-modern and post-structural perspectives also advocate a more radical approach to citizenship. Radical citizenship should be agonistic and antagonistic, allowing for differential conceptions of 'the good', as well as diverse identities and allegiances (Brown, 1997). Radical democracy developed as an alternative concept in the 1960s as a result of increased focus on participation (Heywood, 1992). Drawing parallels from ancient Greek democracy, this approach centres upon 'grass roots democracy' carried out by pressure groups and political activists (Heywood, 1992; Beetham and Boyle, 1998). This perspective on citizenship allows alternative spaces of citizenship to be identified and explored. It is with the consideration of such spaces that chapters 4, 5 and 6 will be concerned.

Cosmopolitan notions of citizenship

Cosmopolitan perspectives argue for a more inclusive and global approach to citizenship. Increased attention on the processes of globalization, regionalization, migration and ecological concerns highlights the significance of cosmopolitan democracy, which displaces democracy tied to the nation-state and instead draws upon a local–global nexus (Lister, 1998; Beck,

2000; Held and McGrew, 2000; McGrew, 2000; Osler, 2005; Osler and Starkey, 2005b). As a result, authors such as Soysal (1994) and Faulks (2000) argue that links between citizenship and the nation-state need to be eroded. As Faulks suggests:

> Cosmopolitan democracy seeks to theorise a citizenship that is global in its orientation and involves not just the protection of rights but also the extension of responsibilities beyond the state and the development of global institutions of governance.

> (2000: 149)

A cosmopolitan approach also regards rights as relational, thus differing from more abstract liberal understandings of rights (Faulks, 2000). According to Faulks global issues such as security and climate change challenge the liberal notion of rights by illustrating that rights can only be maintained if obligations beyond national boundaries are acknowledged. Moreover, processes such as globalization and migration have shifted understandings of belonging to a nation-state and have emphasized plurality in identity. Osler and Starkey (2005b) argue that whilst national understandings obviously remain significant, such global changes are particularly important to acknowledge in relation to devising a citizenship curriculum that is relevant to the lives of contemporary teenagers. Cosmopolitan perspectives, therefore, provide a more inclusive and holistic approach to citizenship. This, Osler and Starkey argue, is important for an increasingly globalized world where, for example, media and communications technology enables people to make connections with others across the globe:

> Cosmopolitan citizenship in a liberal democracy is not an alternative to national citizenship, nor is it even in tension with national citizenship. It is a way of being a citizen at any level, local, national, regional or global. It is based on feelings of solidarity with fellow human beings wherever they are situated.

> (2005b: 23)

Democracy operates at different spatial scales globally. Cosmopolitan citizenship is, therefore, concerned with both national and international issues (Osler and Starkey, 2005b). Held (1995; 1996) calls for the creation of institutions beyond the level of the nation-state, which would exist alongside national institutions. The extent to which globalization has been overstated is the stuff of keen debate as much power remains at the level of the nation-state (Lister, 1997b; 1998; Faulks, 2000). Whilst boundaries have undeniably become more blurred, many have also argued that the world has become more polarized with global trade only benefiting particular areas such as Europe, the USA and Japan (Faulks, 2000).

The growth of the human rights movement and associated international agreements has moved some areas of decision-making beyond the nation-state (Faulks, 2000). Indeed, authors such as Soysal (1994) have argued that the notion of universal human rights replaces the concept of citizenship, whilst others such as Faulks (2000) suggest that citizenship is concerned with political participation and obligations which human rights do not necessarily confer. In critiquing Soysal's (1994) notion that guest-workers in many countries are not citizens but through human rights agreements do benefit from civil and social rights, Faulks (2000) argues that such groups remain excluded from political rights and therefore not able to fully participate. Nevertheless, global conventions on human rights may provide the grounding for a set of common values which could form the basis of cosmopolitan citizenship (Osler and Starkey, 2005b). The importance of the 1989 United Nations Convention on the Rights of the Child (UNCRC) to children's rights and citizenship, therefore, becomes apparent. The UNCRC will be discussed in more detail later in this chapter.

Advocating a cosmopolitan perspective, Osler and Starkey (2005b) suggest that citizenship has three constituent elements: as a status, as a feeling and as a practice. As a status it signifies an individual's relationship with the state. This is often a legal status which affords individuals some rights, and in return expects citizens to fulfil a number of duties. Nevertheless, citizenship may also be regarded as a feeling because individuals may consider themselves to belong to a number of communities, or countries. This is particularly significant in an increasingly globalized world. Osler and Starkey (2005b) argue that a 'sense of belonging' is a prerequisite to a 'sense of citizenship' which highlights the importance of viewing citizenship as more than just a legal status. Finally, they illustrate citizenship as practice whereby individuals or collectives practise active citizenship in a variety of arenas which may or may not include the nation-state.

New feminist perspectives on citizenship

Many feminist writers have strongly criticized dominant conceptualizations of citizenship in that liberal notions in particular espouse universalist principles whilst at the same time exclude, for example, women from different elements (Lister, 1998; Marston and Mitchell, 2004). Many feminist authors have opposed the separation of women to the private sphere and men to the public sphere as exclusionary in terms of women's access to public spaces of citizenship (Painter and Philo, 1995; Foster, 1997; Kjørholt, 2004). Writings on feminist perspectives on citizenship are most eminently associated with the work of Lister (1997a; 1997b; 1998). Lister (1997a; 1997b) argues that citizenship may be exclusive and exclusionary, as well as inclusive. She, therefore, regards inclusion and exclusion as the two constituent elements of citizenship and in a call for an international approach to feminist citizenship theory and practice, she suggests the inclusion/exclusion differential should be viewed as a continuum rather than a dichotomy, as different groups and individuals within society have access to differing levels of meaningful participation (Lister, 1997a). As Lister suggests:

> The boundaries of inclusion and exclusion operate at both a legal and a sociological level through formal and substantive modes of citizenship.
>
> (1998: 53)

In response to more conventional understandings associated with civic republicanism and liberalism Lister (1997b) calls for a 'differentiated universalism' which recognizes particularity. Furthermore, she notes that contemporary understandings of citizenship have progressed from consideration of inclusion and exclusion bounded by the state towards a more holistic approach to both intra-state citizenship and non-residential citizenship. A multi-layered approach to citizenship therefore emerges, encompassing the multiple identities and allegiances individual actors have within society. Like cosmopolitan approaches to citizenship, feminist perspectives also take an internationalist stance uniting the local and the global. In particular, it is at the community level that spaces of citizenship are available to those excluded from more formal political institutions, as Lister suggests:

> It is the local rather than the national which provides the arena for many citizenship struggles of this kind.
>
> (1997b: 33)

For Lister, human agency needs to be central to understandings of citizenship whereby rights become the means through which individuals are able to exert their agency. These rights are fluid and subject to continuous political conflict (Lister, 1997b). Lister therefore proposes a feminist conceptualization of citizenship which synthesizes elements of civic republicanism and liberalism. This alternative notion adapts civic republican citizenship to include women's interests using a broader understanding of the political, which encompasses more radical and oppositional forms of citizenship, for example, protest. Drawing upon the work of Mouffe (1992), Lister calls for a re-conceptualization of citizenship that would:

> draw on both the liberal formulation of free and equal rights-bearing citizens and the richer republican conceptualisation of active political participation and civic engagement (but based on a radical, pluralist reframing of the 'common good').
>
> (Lister, 1997b: 34)

This approach, whilst recognizing that women are active rather than passive agents, also acknowledges the barriers and constraints placed upon women in certain political arenas. Moreover, in these terms citizenship can be viewed as both status and practice:

> To be a citizen, in a sociological sense, means to enjoy the rights necessary for agency and social and political participation. To act as a citizen involves fulfilling the potential of the status. Those who do not fill the potential do not cease to be citizens.
>
> (Lister, 1997b: 36)

Definitions of citizenship also vary between feminists particularly in relation to two key elements of citizenship: rights and duties (Lister, 1997a; Marston and Mitchell, 2004). The social democratic stance, advocated by amongst others Fraser (1997), calls for societal changes which foster equality between men and women in both the public and private arenas. For those on the political Left, 'rights' have often been detrimental to the most socially excluded groups within a liberal democracy (Lister, 1997b). Many on the political Left focus attention on more active elements of citizenship (see Gould, 1988). Moreover, of importance to young teenagers is the exclusion that the duties side of citizenship confers. Duties are often understood by the political Right in terms of contribution to paid employment (Lister, 1997b). Fundamentally, Lister questions how a balance between rights and duties can be fostered for those less powerful in society. She suggests that the synthesis of social rights and political participation is important, in addition to understanding the diverse needs of different social groups within society. In these terms the notion of 'rights' needs to be dynamic (Lister, 1997b).

There are many commonalities between the alternative perspectives on citizenship, all of which provide useful ways of constructing a notion of citizenship which is inclusive for children and young teenagers. This book seeks to promote a more fluid and inclusive approach to citizenship which recognizes the diverse ways in which young teenagers engage in acts of citizenship in a variety of spheres from the conventional to the alternative.

Practical moves towards inclusive citizenship

In line with these alternative conceptualizations there have been a number of practical and/or policy-related measures which offer the potential to alter children and young teenagers' relationship with citizenship. The following section is concerned with the children's rights movement and the development of spaces and opportunities for children's participation as a means of engaging with more social understandings of citizenship.

Children's rights

The children's rights movement has made valuable strides towards upholding the rights of the young across the world, and in a sense has the potential
to facilitate children and young teenagers' access to citizenship. As Osler
and Starkey argue:

> Rights are, nonetheless, the essential starting point for citizenship.
> Rights provide the possibility to practise citizenship and to feel a sense
> of belonging ... children and young people are citizens by virtue of their
> entitlements to rights and their capacity to practise citizenship.
>
> (2005b: 15)

They argue that even if those under eighteen are not entitled to vote they
should be consulted over matters which affect them, although in practice
children and young teenagers are often not viewed as full citizens.

Historically, the greatest movement towards a global human rights
precedent was the signing of the Universal Declaration of Human Rights
by the General Assembly of the United Nations on 10th December 1948
(Steadman, 1998). Consisting of thirty Articles, the Declaration outlined
the standards, freedoms and rights every human should be entitled to in
order to live a just and dignified life, free from prejudice, discrimination,
exploitation and torture. The promotion of this landmark proclamation
was principally to be through schools and other educational institutions
(Steadman, 1998). Integral to the universalization of human rights has
been the development over the past one hundred years of children-specific
rights (PDHRE, 2000). The human rights discourse classifies those under
the age of eighteen as children. Early foundations of the children's rights
movement were formulated through the first Declaration on the Rights of
the Child in 1923 (Muscroft, 1999). Drafted by Eglantyne Jebb, the
Declaration was based upon the belief that child protection was the
responsibility of the whole community, not just the family (Muscroft,
1999). Post-Second World War emphasis on human rights in general
helped foster debate regarding the production of children-specific rights. It
was not, however, until 1959 that the United Nations accepted an
amended draft of Eglantyne Jebb's recommendations. Regrettably, this was
only to be used as a guide rather than legislation to which governments
could be held accountable (Muscroft, 1999). Children's rights, however,
have often been seen to conflict with those of adults in, for example, value
systems associated with 'Victorian' child-rearing (Alexander, 1995;
Muscroft, 1999). These upheld the teaching of morals and responsibility,
the perpetuation of which is best illustrated in the contemporary debate
surrounding smacking, which raises issues not only of protection but civil
rights (Lansdown, 1994).

In the late 1960s children's rights were predominantly centred upon a 'child liberation' standpoint (Hendrick, 1997). Links between the subordination of women and the oppression of children can be identified and outline the need for children's rights to self-determination to be recognized. Notions of vulnerability and protectionism are significant to the development of child-specific rights (Euronet, 2000). Alongside the 'child liberation' discourse, the paternalistic or 'caretaker thesis' emerged, which also acknowledged the marginalization of children (Hendrick, 1997). This approach encapsulated adult protectionist thought and perpetuated the deficit model of childhood (Taylor, 2000). The caretaker thesis is often critiqued for being more aspirational than substantive, and still maintains the assumptions surrounding the nature of the 'best interests' of the child (Hendrick, 1997; O'Brien *et al.*, 2000).

After the 'International Year of the Child' in 1979 the children's rights movement developed greater prominence, and throughout the Cold War years non-governmental organizations (NGOs) played a key role in conceiving the UNCRC (Muscroft, 1999). The adoption of the UNCRC was seen as a mechanism to counter the vulnerable status of children and to recognize state responsibility for parental abuse (Lansdown, 1994), and has been ratified by all but two countries.[7] By 1990 it had become an important part of international law (Muscroft, 1999). Throughout the 1990s, emphasis on the protection of children's rights increased particularly in relation to issues such as trafficking and child labour. Moreover, children and teenagers' participation through mechanisms such as youth councils and forums became a much advocated means of involvement in decision-making (Muscroft, 1999).

The UNCRC consists of fifty-four Articles which relate to four key principles covering: the right to survival and development; respect for a child's best interests; freedom of expression; and anti-discrimination measures. In sum, as Muscroft suggests:

> Children are seen as full human beings, rights-holders who can play an active part in the enjoyment of their rights. They are not – as they have often been presented in the past – mere dependants, the property of their parents. They are not only people who become fully human when they become adults. They are in need of protection but also have strengths. Every child is seen as important, no matter what its abilities, origin or gender. Their views and opinions are significant.
>
> (1999: 16)

Concurrently, global movements such as the UNCRC go some way to provide children and teenagers with a degree of participation. Sangha (2001) suggests that the UNCRC is indeed compatible with Marshall's (1950) definition of citizenship. To reinforce this Muscroft notes one of the principal ideas of the UNCRC:

Children are seen as active members of their local communities and national societies. They contribute their labour to a variety of work and care responsibilities inside and outside the home. They play an important part in cultural and leisure activities in and out of school. They are interested in what is going on around them, especially that which affects them directly. If encouraged they become active and involved citizens.

(1999: 17)

Within this context, Lister's (1997a) notions of the inclusivity and exclusivity of citizenship may be more appropriate to consider.

Nevertheless, the implementation of the UNCRC has been both sporadic and problematic for it exists within a framework of wider political difficulties and changes. The 1990s were marked by the end of the Cold War and the dominance of global free-market capitalism. Such economic shifts have increased inequalities within and between nations, impacting greatly upon the lives of many children. Globally, well over half of those living in poverty are children, many millions of whom do not live to see their fifth birthday, or are forced to work in exploitative conditions or who lack access to education, sanitation or food (Muscroft, 1999). The UNCRC has been integral to raising awareness of children's needs in a multitude of environments, thereby ensuring that many children are treated with dignity, and that children's voices are placed on policy agendas. The period prior to and during the development of the UNCRC has witnessed both an increase in and the growth of organizations working on behalf of children's rights and countering abuse, as well as children-led movements (Muscroft, 1999).

Both Conservative and Labour Governments in the UK have constructed complicated and often contradictory responses to children's rights and the UNCRC. Positive reactions have included numerous developments such as the abolition of corporal punishment in schools and children's homes in 1986; the establishment of the Children's Rights Development Unit in 1992 (Hendrick, 1997); the 'Children and Young People's Unit' in 2000 (CYPU, 2001; Klaushofer, 2002); the Government Green Paper *Every Child Matters* in 2003 (DfES, 2003); and the appointment of a Minister for Children in 2003 (BBC, 2003a). Adversely, policy decisions such as the Crime and Disorder Act 1998 have given local authorities the power to impose curfews on children under the age of ten and little has been done to outlaw corporal punishment by parents (Muscroft, 1999). These issues raise questions regarding the UK's commitment to children's rights. Furthermore, the debate surrounding the rights of children is thrown into disarray by determining what constitutes a child. The UNCRC states that children are those under the age of eighteen unless an individual nation has a younger franchise. Nevertheless, many children and teenagers have actively challenged notions of childhood in both positive and negative ways. One more positive example is the Gillick case in 1983 in which a mother lost her battle against the legal system to prohibit the medical profession from prescribing contraceptives to children under the age of sixteen without parental consent (Valentine, 1999; BBC, 2003b). By 1984 the Gillick Judgment was established which stated that:

> in the absence of an express statutory rule, all parental authority 'yields to the child's right to make his [sic] own decisions when he reaches a sufficient understanding and intelligence to be capable of making up his own mind on the matter requiring decision'.
>
> (Keele, 2003: webpage)

Alternatively a negative example of the way children have challenged 'childhood' is the Bulger Case. In 1993 two boys aged ten were imprisoned for the murder of toddler James Bulger. Whilst the UNCRC has been significant in creating a children's rights dialogue amongst national governments and organizations such as NGOs, the extent to which it has been promoted and received by adults and children is both questionable and difficult to measure.

Whilst child-specific rights may have the potential for the empowerment of children and young people, it must be questioned whether such an approach could ultimately result in the reinforcement of the adult/child dichotomy, constructing children as vulnerable and assigning childhood as a right itself (Taylor, 2000). The development of such rights, by the adult world, may ultimately seek to maintain children as 'other', much like a denizen or occupant of a community who is admitted only certain rights. Nevertheless, Osler and Starkey (2005b) argue that the UNCRC is a positive step in promoting young people's citizenship because the almost global ratification means that the majority of countries have a duty to uphold the 54 Articles. Not only has the UNCRC been important in supporting child protection issues, but it has also been significant in promoting the notion of children's rights and has encouraged policy-makers to include children and young teenagers in decision-making over issues which affect their lives, as well as service provision. This is, therefore, an important means of affording children and young teenagers the rights of citizenship (Osler and Starkey, 2005b).

Opportunities for participation

Opportunities for children's participation in some elements of contemporary society are a relatively recent phenomenon. As James and James (2004) highlight it was not until the 1989 Children Act that the common adage 'children should be seen and not heard' was challenged. Such moves have, therefore, changed the way childhood is viewed.

Article 12 of the UNCRC stresses the fundamental need for children's opinions to be considered:

Parties shall assure to the child who is capable of forming his or her own views the right to express those views freely in all matters affecting the child, the views of the child being given due weight in accordance with the age and maturity of the child.

(United Nations, 1990)

Despite the ethos of the UNCRC, there was initial reluctance by many professionals to acknowledge the value of consulting those too young to vote (Muscroft, 1999). Nevertheless, many countries have created proactive, coordinated methods of participation for children and teenagers. 'Association Nationale des Conseils d'Enfants et de Jeunes' in France, for example, aims to develop participation at an early age through town councils (Jodry, 1997). More broadly, current debates include the introduction of a European Union Youth Policy (CYPU, 2002). In the UK, the Children and Young People's Unit has a Youth Advisory Forum (CYPU, 2002). Government policies such as 'Sure Start' and 'Connexions' have also acknowledged that social exclusion affects children and teenagers (see Inman, 1999; Literacy Trust, 2001; Sure Start, 2002; Countryside Agency, 2003b), although 'Sure Start' explicitly supported the parents of young children. The government has adopted some consultation strategies, for example, young people were invited to comment upon the Government Green Paper *Every Child Matters*. Numerous youth councils, forums and parliaments have also emerged providing children and teenagers with opportunities to participate in some contexts (Matthews and Limb, 1998; Wainwright, 2001). Horelli (1998) illustrates children's participation in planning 'child-friendly' environments, drawing on examples from Finland, Switzerland and France, and he concludes by calling for a redefinition of agency in the context of increased children's participation. Furthermore, Alanen states that children should be viewed as 'agents of their own lives in a new paradigm of socialisation' (1997: 251).

This move towards promoting children and young people's participation has led to a distinct set of political institutions outside of the adult realm and arguably superficial. Children and young people are merely afforded the status of 'taking part' (Hart, 1992; 1997; Wellard *et al.*, 1997), as full participation is frequently regarded as a threat to adult autonomy. Ideological barriers exist in relation to how 'childhood' and 'youth' are characterized as incompetent and irresponsible (Lansdown, 1995). Participation, therefore, remains constructed as an 'adult' activity, carried out in 'adult' institutions, and perhaps, more fundamentally, seldom results in any real action (Oakley, 1994). The notion of participation, however, remains regarded as beneficial to children, teenagers, parents and wider society, allowing expression, mutual respect, conflict resolution and the improvement of democratic procedures (Miller, 1996).

What is most apparent is that whilst attention has begun to focus on fostering children and teenagers' participation, this is often within the context of specifically children-centred processes, such as youth forums. Although such attention is fundamentally important, debate must be (re)centred upon broader issues of exclusion from citizenship and belonging in order to acknowledge the frustrations felt by teenagers at their lack of participatory opportunities, and also, conversely, the actions that teenagers take to reshape their communities. Moreover, Osler and Starkey (2005b) argue that it is important that the obligations of the UNCRC are fully recognized and that children and young teenagers are meaningfully consulted on matters of concern to them as a principle and as a requirement of the UNCRC. Whilst many important moves have been made within the UK to involve children and young teenagers politically an important shift is still needed in how young people are meaningfully included as citizens. Osler and Starkey (2005b) advocate legislation as one way to alter the dominant political culture.

The next step for teenagers' citizenship

Reflecting upon the opening paragraphs of chapters 1 and 2 – the 'pupil protests' against military action in Iraq – children and young teenagers, by virtue of their age and societal positioning, inhabit a challenging and contradictory relationship with citizenship. Cockburn (1998) calls for citizenship that respects difference and includes all children, placing them as integral members of society, rather than as apprentices. This requires a societal shift from rights-based rhetoric towards recognition, not only of children and teenagers' competencies, but of the interdependence of all groups within society, particularly in relation to citizenship (Cockburn, 1998; Roche, 1999). Without such empowerment, children and teenagers are confined to exercise power through the 'symbolic politics of protest' (Roche, 1999) and so risk labels of 'deviant youth'. Analysis of children and teenagers' citizenship must, therefore, transcend ideas relating to passive bearers of rights and move towards an understanding based upon the abilities of children and teenagers to (re)shape environments (Helve and Wallace, 2001).

This book, in drawing upon more contemporary and alternative understandings of citizenship, advocates Marston and Mitchell's (2004) notion of 'citizenship formation' which recognizes citizenship as constantly in a state of flux particularly in terms of its relationship with the nation-state. The arguments presented also draw upon more cultural and social understandings of citizenship which include moves towards young people's participation whilst retaining the importance of conventional political theories in shaping both teenagers' spaces of and opportunities for citizenship. Dillabough and Arnot assert:

It is time to change the ways in which we struggle for democracy in education – to abandon the 'lion's skin' and construct new definitions of citizenship which are based upon the needs of contemporary women.

(2000: 38)

A similar approach is required to enhance the status of teenagers. Following this call, the arguments presented in this book are framed by an understanding that citizenship needs to be elastic, fluid and most of all inclusive. I also promote a more explicit spatialized analysis of citizenship that explores the complexities of space and place; an analysis that seeks to understand the struggles, challenges and conflicts inherent in the acts of citizenship which occur in these arenas. As chapters 4, 5 and 6 will highlight, micro-spaces of citizenship *matter* and reveal much about teenagers' abilities and opportunities to act as citizens. At the global or macro-level citizenship also *matters* to teenagers as many have an important relationship with global citizenship through disparate means from consumerism to protest, through the internet, sport and the media and via diasporic identities. Alternative understandings of citizenship which draw upon more cosmopolitan and feminist perspectives are particularly important for young teenagers for it is at the mezzo-level of the nation-state, the arena which so fundamentally matters in terms of conventional understandings of citizenship, that the real challenges lie. Akin to other sections of the population, many teenagers are sceptical about state-based politics and politicians (ESRC, 2005) and remain excluded from many mainstream political institutions by virtue of their age. This is not to disregard the important consultations that have been carried out with young people, but to acknowledge that there is still a long way to go until the majority of young people have been afforded meaningful opportunities for participation. The next chapter is concerned with the development of citizenship education as one means of (re)defining teenagers' relationship with citizenship.

Chapter 3

Actively learning citizenship

Introducing education for citizenship

Young teenagers have a problematic relationship with citizenship and within the context of many dominant understandings the young are predominantly defined as citizens-in-the-making who need to learn how to affectively participate in Western democracy. Within England concerns about teenage apathy, anti-social behaviour and a more general decline in interest in formal politics have undoubtedly fuelled concerns about engagement in democratic institutions and processes, exacerbating the need for a more coherent and solid foundation for the teaching of citizenship in schools. This chapter represents the first of two explicitly concerned with teenagers' citizenship within school. Young people spend a significant and increasing proportion of their time at school: a place where conventionally children and teenagers have had little opportunity to voice their opinions, and arguably one arena in which adults exert significantly more power and control. The spaces occupied by teenagers within school are highly structured, controlled and disciplined (Holloway and Valentine, 2000b), and to some degree the classroom environment and didactic style of teaching has changed little over the past century (Osler and Starkey, 2005b). In recent years there have been a number of significant moves towards listening to and promoting the voices of young people within school, from young children in the early years of primary school through to students in the sixth form and college. Policy initiatives such as the introduction of citizenship education and *Every Child Matters* (DfES, 2003) seek to promote participation and involvement in the hope that such moves will engage the young within school and beyond.

In England citizenship education became compulsory for children and teenagers in secondary education in September 2002. This new wave of teaching democracy is seen as a distinct shift from the civics education of the 1960s and 1970s to that based upon discussion and participation. This chapter begins by detailing the context in which citizenship education became compulsory, outlining how the subject in its current guise differs from past teachings. Subsequently, the chapter examines the development of the curriculum focusing on the findings of the Advisory Group on *Education for Citizenship and the Teaching of Democracy in Schools* and the Citizenship Order. Finally, the chapter draws together findings from this study and the research of others to evaluate the conceptual underpinnings of the citizenship curriculum, the implementation of the subject, and importantly, young teenagers' preliminary reactions to compulsory citizenship education.

Contextualizing contemporary citizenship education

The principal stimuli for the introduction of compulsory citizenship education may be divided into three broad categories. First, the historical context leading up to the introduction of the subject is important for understanding the development of such education in England. Second, policy concerns relating to apathy and political disengagement are one of the key driving forces for introducing a curriculum based upon active citizenship. Finally, there is the rationale for implementing a common citizenship that is both flexible and to some degree prescriptive. I examine each category here.

An historical perspective

Political or citizenship education is not new and civic education was advocated in France as early as the late eighteenth century. Heater (2001) cites the 1763 publication *Essai d'Education Nationale* as an example of this. In England, citizenship education has had a variety of foci, although generally it has been afforded sparse attention. A number of factors, identified by Heater (2001) as political, social and pedagogic, have been regarded as the key determinants in accounting for the low priority bestowed on civics or citizenship education. Lister *et al.* (2001) suggest that government fears about political indoctrination have, in part, fuelled inertia. Taking an historical perspective, Heater (2001) argues that issues of democracy in Britain and more general apathy towards formal politics; class divisions both within society and the education system; and a lack of guidance for teachers, coupled with the fear that young people may well be indoctrinated have resulted in little emphasis on citizenship in formal education.

The work of economist A.H. Marshall was significant in the late 1800s in England as his writings on the working classes advocated state education as a basic right (Dwyer, 2004). Later motivations for the introduction of public schooling placed emphasis on creating an educated workforce to sustain capitalism and to foster 'future responsible citizens' (Isin and Wood, 1999). Victorian industrialists such as Lord Leverhulme insisted on compulsory citizenship lessons for his workers as an integral part of moral education (Duffy,

1996; Heater, 2001). The extension of the franchise in 1867 (and 1970) brought to the fore concerns about citizen competency. As a result politicians became concerned about the abilities of the electorate to make informed decisions (Heater, 2001). In the post-Victorian period English civics education did develop to some degree with both the First and Second World Wars focusing attention on world citizenship (Edwards and Fogelman, 1991; Heater, 2001; see also Grosvenor and Lawn, 2004). Britain's role in the world during times of global conflict, and the decline of the empire had a significant influence on the attention given to civic and political education. During the 1940s the government made several positive steps towards introducing citizenship education with, for example, the publication of *Citizens Growing Up* in 1949. Conflict amongst politicians at that time meant that the subject was again sidelined, although (non-controversial) elements were taught through more traditional subjects (Heater, 2001).

By the 1950s and 1960s, citizenship education had become relegated and few policy documents were produced, which implies that little attention was afforded to the subject. Notable and relatively influential exceptions included the *Schools Council Working Paper* which argued the case for political education, and more significantly believed that young people were capable of understanding political issues (Heater, 2001). During the 1970s and 1980s opposition remained to the notion of citizenship education and debate was interlaced with conflict over the most appropriate place for learning citizenship. During the late 1980s, research on the feasibility of a proposed policy relating to voluntary community service was undertaken in order to engage teenagers with the then relatively unfamiliar term, 'citizenship'. Whilst in the feasibility study participants' opinions relating to what it means to be a citizen were diverse, there was much consensus on the need for citizenship education in schools, especially in the final two years of compulsory education (Richardson, 1990; Weller, 2003). It was not until the 1990s that civics or political education was referred to as citizenship education; the former term conferring notions of compliance and submission (Heater, 2001). Debate over the most suitable arena to learn citizenship finally culminated in the 1996 Education Act which legislated for the political impartiality of schools and staff. Importantly in 1988 citizenship became one of five cross-curricula themes (Biesta and Lawy, 2006), and in 1999 the Department for Education and Employment (DfEE) made positive steps towards the implementation of statutory citizenship education (Heater, 2001). From September 2002, citizenship education became compulsory for children and teenagers at Key Stages 3 and 4 (aged 11–16) in England (Lawton *et al.*, 2000; Biesta and Lawy, 2006). This new wave of teaching citizenship is regarded as markedly different from earlier civics education (Kingston, 2002; Wolchover, 2002).

Contemporary policy concerns

It is apparent that in historical terms the economic, social and political context of the country has had a significant influence on the emphasis and direction afforded to civics or citizenship education. In many ways this development in education policy has, for many decades, been an 'unfinished project' within Britain, and it is within the context of the contemporary political climate that the 'project' has become consolidated. For the current government the underlying rationale of contemporary citizenship education lies with reducing voter apathy, countering alienation and providing a unifying element to social exclusion policy (Bright and Dodd, 1998; Crick, 2000; Lister *et al.*, 2001; Leighton, 2004). Otherwise known as the 'democratic deficit', concerns about the impact of widespread political disengagement on democracy are central to this perceived 'crisis' (Kerr, 1999a; Cunningham and Lavalette, 2004). Crick (2000) argues that the introduction of the subject has been, for many countries, a response to a crisis or event. Indeed, several authors have argued that the current government's enthusiasm for citizenship education is part of an international resurgence in interest following the 'democratization' of former communist states, and a decrease in the engagement of the populace in formal politics in more liberal states (Halpern *et al.*, 2002; Biesta and Lawy, 2006). Many countries in the Western world now teach citizenship in schools. Fears relating to disengagement in formal politics and the preservation of democracy have, therefore, fuelled drives towards citizenship education as a means of motivating the populace (Biesta and Lawy, 2006).

As alluded to in chapter 2, growing concern about voter apathy is frequently targeted at the young, and the current New Labour Government continues to pursue policies which focus upon the political engagement of young people despite a plethora of studies which produce inconsistent findings on teenage apathy (Biesta and Lawy, 2006). Flew (2000) draws together a number of reports, some of which suggest that those aged 18–24 are not necessarily less engaged than other age groups and indeed it is only the middle-aged cohort that are significantly more engaged in conventional electoral politics than other groups. Flew argues that there is some evidence of disaffection amongst young people in relation to formal party politics. But all too often political apathy has been read as synonymous with declining interest in party politics, for as Cunningham and Lavalette (2004) note, many young people *are* actively engaged in other political groups, movements and campaigns.

The introduction of compulsory citizenship education has also arisen amidst growing concerns regarding (anti-social) behaviour amongst children and young teenagers (Faulks, 2006). Such fears have resulted in calls for the teaching of social and moral responsibility, and the training of 'future responsible citizens'. For as Bernard Weatherill, the then Speaker of the House of Commons, stated in his forward to the Commission on Citizenship's (1990) report *Encouraging Citizenship*:

> I believe that citizenship, like anything else, has to be learned. Young people do not become good citizens by accident more than they become good nurses or good engineers or good bus drivers or computer scientists. My concern [is] whether we offer enough encouragement to our young people to learn how to be good citizens.

The drive for contemporary citizenship education is, therefore, a response to a perceived crisis in democracy, and in particular the apathy and behaviour of the young.

A centralized approach to citizenship

Whilst citizenship and/or civics education has a long-established history in the USA and in many European countries little emphasis has been placed on the subject in England. Although citizenship has been present within the curriculum, provision has been patchy and ill-defined. One of the key reasons for the introduction of *compulsory* citizenship education, rather than maintaining citizenship as a cross-curricula theme, was to provide a more consistent and explicit education on citizenship and democracy (Kerr, 1999a). Prior to the compulsory introduction of the subject many schools in England taught aspects of citizenship under the auspices of lessons such as geography, history and religious education. Related topic areas were also delivered though Personal, Social and Health Education (PSHE). In these terms citizenship was an implicit part of the curriculum and schools varied considerably in their emphasis and coverage of the subject. This approach was not deemed to be effective in training a nation of young citizens-in-the-making. Despite concerns regarding the disparate provision of citizenship education prior to 2002, Halpern *et al.* (2002), in their study of Hertfordshire schools in 2000, suggest that citizenship was perhaps more commonly studied than other research has implied. Whilst they acknowledge that the introduction of citizenship as a cross-curricula theme may have had some bearing on their findings, many schools were engaged in both teaching and practising some aspects of citizenship prior to September 2002. Nevertheless, the current government regards statutory citizenship as necessary for ensuring that all young people achieve sufficient knowledge and skills in the workings of democracy.

Historical developments, policy pressures and the drive towards centralizing and universalizing the curriculum may be regarded as the key contexts in which citizenship education became compulsory in England. The central assumption by government is that citizenship education is a 'good thing' which will result in the strengthening of democracy. The teaching of citizenship is not, however, necessarily synonymous with creating 'good citizens' (Leighton, 2004; Watts, 2006).

Introducing contemporary citizenship education

It is important to examine the decision-making processes behind the formulation of contemporary citizenship education, such as the recommendations of the Advisory Group on *Education for Citizenship and the Teaching of Democracy in Schools* and the Citizenship Order, in order to understand the ways in which current policy relates to teenagers' status as citizens.

Policy and the Crick Report

In 1997 David Blunkett, the then Secretary of State for Education and Employment, published *Excellence in Schools*; a White Paper (DfEE, 1997) which, in part, argued that the teaching of citizenship and democracy should be reinforced within schools. As a result of the paper, an Advisory Group on *Education for Citizenship and the Teaching of Democracy in Schools* (hereafter, Advisory Group) was established (Kerr, 1999a; Nelson and Kerr, 2005; Biesta and Lawy, 2006). Chaired by Professor Bernard Crick and managed by the Qualifications and Curriculum Authority (QCA), the Advisory Group consisted of 'non-partisan' representatives from a number of schools, academia, local authorities, the media, political think-tanks and other NGOs, such as the Citizenship Foundation and the Church of England. The role of the Advisory Group was to determine the aim of citizenship education, the shape and purpose of the citizenship curriculum and to assess how schools might engage in practices of good citizenship (Flew, 2000). The Advisory Group made a series of key recommendations suggesting that citizenship in schools was so essential that a statutory Order was necessary (see also Kerr, 1999a):

> We unanimously advise the Secretary of State that citizenship and the teaching of democracy, construed in a broad sense ... is so important both for schools and the life of the nation that there must be a statutory requirement on schools to ensure that it is part of the entitlement of all pupils. It can no longer sensibly be left to uncoordinated local initiatives which vary greatly in number, content and method. This is an inadequate basis for animating the idea of a common citizenship with democratic values.
>
> (QCA, 1998: 7)

The Advisory Group believed that the advantages of statutory citizenship education would be wide-ranging: motivating young people to participate as informed responsible citizens; guiding teachers towards a more consistent education for citizenship; encouraging schools to foster an effective curriculum and links to the local community; as well as benefits for wider society (QCA, 1998). As a result of the Advisory Group's recommendations citizenship education became a compulsory element of the curriculum at Key Stages 3 and 4, and also became an entitlement for those aged 16–19 (Kerr, 1999a; DfEE, 2000; CYPU, 2002; Nelson and Kerr, 2005).

Findings from the Advisory Group were published in several phases concluding in September 1998 with *Education for Citizenship and the Teaching of Democracy in Schools*, commonly referred to as the 'Crick Report' (QCA, 1998). The fundamental aim of citizenship education outlined in the Crick Report was 'active citizenship', and much focus was placed upon the importance of community involvement in strengthening the outcomes of such education (QCA, 1998; Chisholm, 2001). The Advisory Group drew heavily upon T.H. Marshall's notion of citizenship, arguing that active citizenship should be defined by the interaction between Marshall's (1950) three elements of citizenship, political, civil and social rights, and should not focus upon one at the expense of another (QCA, 1998; Kerr, 1999a; Crick, 2000; Wragg, 2002; Biesta and Lawy, 2006). This notion of 'active citizenship' drew upon and challenged the proposals of the Conservative Government in the 1980s who associated citizenship with good behaviour (Hall *et al.*, 1999; Crick, 2000). Contemporary focus is primarily centred upon a state-based understanding of citizenship and a concern to re-engage citizens with the government against a perceived tide of apathy and disengagement (QCA, 1998; Jochum *et al.*, 2005; Biesta and Lawy, 2006). In Crick's own vision of citizenship, involvement, voluntary work, assisting neighbours and so on should be done by an individual on an entirely voluntary basis. With particular regard to citizenship education active citizens should be trained to act freely, although this may have unseen and challenging connotations for the government. As Crick argues:

> If we teach to induce the correct substantive attitudes (whether 'respect for the rule of law', 'proper individualism', 'the classless society', or whatever), it is not politics or citizenship we are teaching: it is something at best paternally approved, our quasi-autocratic friend, the 'good citizen', say rather 'good subject'.
>
> (2000: 106)

The Advisory Group recommended three foci for the new curriculum comprising social and moral responsibility, 'helpful involvement' in the community, and political literacy (Kerr, 1999a; Crick, 2000; Biesta and Lawy, 2006; Ireland *et al.*, 2006a). Importantly, the emphasis of the Crick Report was not just upon knowledge but upon developing understanding within school, and within the wider community. More recently, research by Ireland *et al.* (2006a) suggests that there has been a move towards focusing upon the three 'Cs' of citizenship as a more appropriate (re)conceptualization relevant to the everyday needs of practitioners. The three 'Cs' include: learning citizenship in lessons, active citizenship in school, and active citizenship outside school. The Citizenship Foundation (2000) also suggests that, in practice, citizenship education can be approached from two levels. The first involves education relating to issues in fairness, democracy and identity, in addition to debates concerning moral dilemmas, whilst a broader approach to issues, such as sustainable development, globalization, poverty and human rights, is given to the second focus concerning global citizenship.

Constituting 5 per cent of curriculum time the key focus of the subject is upon learning outcomes rather than a prescriptive schedule of work (Kerr, 1999a; Crick, 2000; Clemitshaw and Calvert, 2005). Lessons in citizenship are unique in that schools have some flexibility over subject matter and timetabling (Kerr et al., 2003). In 1999, secondary schools in England were given two years to prepare for statutory citizenship classes and could opt for one of three approaches. The first involved incorporating citizenship education within the PSHE curriculum. In a later evaluation OFSTED (2003) discovered that this approach was often ineffective as young people were not always aware they were studying the subject, and because 'citizenship' was not adequately emphasized. The second option placed citizenship within other national curriculum subjects and was also problematic. Even if a citizenship-related topic had been covered in history or geography, it was not always covered in a way that sufficiently extracted themes of citizenship. This approach was only effective if the citizenship element was made explicit. The most effective means of implementing the subject, OFSTED (2003) suggest, is through distinct, regular lessons labelled 'citizenship' as well as through other curriculum subjects.

The Citizenship Order prescribed that at Key Stages 3 and 4 the curriculum should provide students with the knowledge and skills to become informed citizens (Ireland et al., 2006a; 2006b; see also Crick 2002). The areas studied at Key Stage 3 include: legal and human rights; national, regional, religious and ethnic identities; the role of local and central government; the role of parliament; the electoral system and voting; the role of voluntary groups; conflict resolution; the role of the media in society; and the world as a global community. Similar areas are strengthened at Key Stage 4 alongside additional topics such as: participation in democratic processes; the economy; the rights and responsibilities of consumers and employers; and the role of the UK in the EU. The curriculum guidelines suggest that citizenship education will help young people to develop a number of skills, improving their communication, IT, teamwork, problem-solving and entrepreneurial skills (DfEE and QCA, 1999; QCA, 2000; DfES, 2006).

Today citizenship education is, in many ways, a much more explicit element of the curriculum, although it has not been introduced without controversy. Indeed, some head teachers and policy-makers felt that citizenship did not need to be taught as it already resonated through the ethos of a 'good school'. Furthermore, whilst the curriculum content appears flexible it is prescriptive in the sense that it imposes one particular understanding of citizenship onto the framework of the curriculum. It is to the evaluation of contemporary citizenship education that this chapter now turns.

Evaluating citizenship education conceptually

An analysis of the concepts and assumptions underlying the current curriculum highlights three problematic areas: namely, the conceptualization of childhood; definitions of 'citizenship' and 'politics'; and understandings of identity.

Re-constructing childhood?

Prior to the introduction of compulsory citizenship education citizenship-related issues were presented through the notion of the 'professional pupil': a student who knew how to behave appropriately and considerately (Gordon et al., 2000). Writing before September 2002, Wyness (2000) viewed the curriculum development with relative optimism, arguing that more recent educational reforms such as citizenship education have the potential to challenge the way childhood is viewed. For example, the Crick Report brought to the fore a number of key issues relating to children's competency, including its emphasis on the importance of making citizenship relevant to both young people's present lives and their future roles, in addition to its focus on active involvement in the community and at school; seemingly positive moves for children's status.

Since September 2002 authors such as James and James (2004) have been far more critical with regard to the effect of citizenship education on young people's status within society. For example, children and young teenagers continue to be regarded as non-citizens. Biesta and Lawy argue:

> As long as citizenship is conceived of as an outcome, it places young people in the problematic position of not-yet-being-a-citizen.
>
> (2006: 72)

A number of problems are, therefore, apparent in the way young people have been construed. First, the citizenship curriculum focuses upon the training of individuals, in essence accrediting blame to individual young people for social problems and political apathy. Second, the curriculum focuses upon a particular kind of social and moral responsibility which does not appear to provide teenagers with the opportunity to challenge the status quo. Rather, it is more concerned with instilling a sense of respect for authority, for example, to become 'helpfully involved in the life and concerns of their school and local communities' (Crick, 2000: 9). Whilst Crick (2000) believes that a degree of scepticism (but not cynicism) towards the government is healthy, much of the ethos of the curriculum is about compliance:

> The agency of children, it would seem, is perceived to be too risky to allow them to be citizens – even within their space of the school.
>
> (James and James, 2004: 134)

Authors such as Brighouse (1998) argue that civic/citizenship education must involve critical analysis in order to uphold citizen autonomy, and yet it appears that the current curriculum seeks to curtail non-conformity. Indeed, for citizenship education to effectively respond to the government's concerns, young people must comply with more conventional understandings of political participation.

Finally, there is an underlying assumption that teenagers need training and encouragement in practising and learning citizenship within school and their local communities. Whilst to some extent this may be the case, sparse attention is given to recognizing the contributions that many teenagers already make to their schools and communities. Incorporating these acts of engagement into the curriculum, so that teenagers can share ideas and learn from the experiences of friends and peers, is essential. The neglect of teenagers' current involvement is a prime illustration of how policy shapes the construction of childhood rendering the young as citizens-in-the-making (James and James, 2004). Policy-makers afford little attention to the agency of children and teenagers in ensuring/constraining the 'success' of different policy initiatives. It is indeed ironic and perhaps short-sighted that membership of the Advisory Group did not include children and teenagers for it is young people themselves who are likely to determine whether the outcomes of the curriculum match the government's expectations.

Problematic definitions

Contemporary citizenship education may also be criticized for the rigid definition of 'citizenship' employed (Faulks, 2006; see also Gordon *et al.*, 2000). This understanding equates citizenship with state-based politics which does not adequately address the role and place of the global citizen. Crick does critique the 'political literacy' lessons of the 1970s for utilizing a narrow definition of 'the political' which did not acknowledge political literacy learnt from small group membership (Crick, 2000). Nevertheless, the Crick Report, whilst acknowledging young people's involvement in single issue groups and political campaigns, maintains a vision of citizenship based upon participation in formal democratic structures, and indeed arguably dismisses other forms of engagement (see QCA, 1998). This is, perhaps, hardly surprising when many of the key figures of the Advisory Group are members of institutions and organizations (educational, religious and parliamentary) most likely to be fearful of a lack of engagement in formal politics, and it appears that children and teenagers were not directly consulted with regard to the content of the curriculum. Based on evidence from their study with young people aged 16–22, Lister *et al.* (2001) argue that a broad definition of 'the political' is needed for effective citizenship education.

It is fruitful to draw upon Blaug's (2002) notions of 'incumbent' and 'critical' democracy to understand the key difficulties inherent in the citizenship curriculum. 'Incumbent' democracy, as Watts (2006) suggests, denotes the kind of compliance with the government expressed in the Crick Report, whilst 'critical' democracy refers to alternative forms of citizenship which encompass struggles and protest and may be in opposition to the government (Faulks, 2006). This mirrors Lister's (1998) argument that active citizenship can be more grass-roots-based and more radical than is conceived of in the current curriculum. As Watts (2006) argues, the political actions of many young people may be regarded within the realms of 'critical democracy' and have, therefore, essentially been disregarded, for example, participating in pressure groups is not viewed by the Advisory Group as political.

Definitions of 'politics' inevitably change over time and mean different things within different contexts, for example, post-war understandings often focused on political institutions whereas more recent understandings also include social movements, for example, the animal rights movement (Faulks, 2006). The student protests against the war in Iraq in 2003 provide a useful example of the contradictions inherent in citizenship education in its current form. As Cunningham and Lavalette (2004) discuss, citizenship education as outlined by Crick and colleagues did move away from traditional understandings of civics education to highlight the importance of fostering 'active citizenship'. This inevitably creates tensions within a curriculum that simultaneously attempts to reinforce compliance and uphold social order, as well as support young people to challenge the status quo (Cunningham and Lavalette, 2004). Cunningham and Lavalette (2004) do not believe that citizenship education influenced young people's decisions to protest. It is, nevertheless, paradoxical that their actions were not regarded as a legitimate form of active citizenry that could be constructively drawn upon, discussed and analysed within the classroom.

Duffy (1996) provides a further critique of citizenship education's focus on creating 'good citizens' by questioning the ambiguities inherent in what it is to be, and what one must do and accept, to be a 'good citizen'. The Commission on Citizenship's (1990) consultative research with young adults revealed that, for many, citizenship encompassed feelings of belonging resulting from either national identity or conforming to laws and entitlement to rights. Such complexities relating to citizenship are by no means contemporary. Duffy (1996), for example, places particular emphasis on Aristotelian notions surrounding lack of agreement on definitions of citizenship. This, Duffy (1996) suggests, is particularly prominent in Britain today during a period of globalization and devolution.

Citizenship for cosmopolitan Britain

Finally, the construction of citizen identity within the current curriculum raises a number of problematic issues. Whilst the curriculum does, to some degree, focus on global issues, religious and ethnic identities and multiculturalism, the language of the National Curriculum more generally promotes a particular set of values which comprise an Anglo-centric, Christian, heterosexual citizen. This, Leighton (2004) rightly argues, does not represent an inclusive notion of citizenship. Moreover, the Crick Report also states that the majority population should respect and tolerate minority groups whilst at the same time minority groups have to go one step further by assimilating towards a common citizenship which is inherently bound to Britishness. Viewing citizenship as an integral part of British identity, the government appears to utilize an unclear definition of citizenship tied to the problematic notion of Britishness (Bhattacharyya, 2004). Indeed, Gifford (2004) argues that part of the premise for citizenship education lies in the restoration of national citizenship. The marriage between nationality and citizenship or 'ethnic multiculturalism', emphasized in the Crick Report, does not provide space for multiple identities, instead assuming that citizens are members of a single nation-state. Moreover, 'ethnic multiculturalism' does not recognize diversity within groups (Faulks, 2006). In these terms, diversity is arguably viewed as a problem rather than a positive dimension of society. Furthermore, valuable work by Osler and Starkey (2005b) highlights the lack of emphasis on racism and inequality within the Crick Report. This, they argue, is institutional racism. Faulks offers an alternative perspective, 'civic multiculturalism', which regards nationality and citizenship as mutually exclusive:

> A healthy multicultural society will, then, constantly modify its associated forms of citizenship through dialogue and democratic interaction that cross social and cultural boundaries.
>
> (2006: 63)

Citizenship education needs to have a more fluid idea of identity, and to explore issues of equality and inequality. Moreover, inequalities and a lack of equality of opportunity for many minority ethnic groups have serious implications for levels of active citizenship (Faulks, 2006).

There have been a number of initiatives, conferences and discussions, including the 'international consensus panel on education for global citizenship in contexts of diversity' in 2003, which have sought to develop a more cosmopolitan approach to citizenship education in recognition that many young people are 'growing up' in multicultural contexts, as well as in an increasingly globalized world (Osler, 2005). The focus on issues of multi-culturalism is of great importance, although it is beyond the realms of this book to fully engage in this aspect of the debate in its reflection of the experiences of teenagers growing up in a predominantly white, rural area of England. The work of authors such as Osler and Starkey, however, highlight the shortcomings of citizenship education in this respect, in addition to promoting the need for a more cosmopolitan notion of citizenship (Osler, 2005; Osler and Starkey, 2001; 2005b).

Fundamentally, Duffy (1996) warns that citizenship education cannot compensate for more structural inequalities, and that for such education to be 'effective' the world outside of educational institutions needs to provide spaces for children's (and teenagers') citizenship. Hart (1992) also argues that education on democracy is fundamental, suggesting that participation cannot be taught as an abstraction but only through praxis (see also Alderson, 2000b).

Evaluating citizenship education in praxis

A number of studies have evaluated the worth and success of citizenship education to date (see, for example, Kerr *et al.*, 2003; 2004; OFSTED, 2003; Faulks, 2006). Many have found great confusion amongst teachers and a general feeling amongst educational organizations that citizenship education, in its current guise, has not been successfully implemented. Thus it is important to explore the development of a common citizenship, teachers' perspectives and teenagers' preliminary thoughts during the introduction of the subject. This exploration serves as a precursor to more general discussion of citizenship in praxis in schools in the next chapter.

A common citizenship?

One of the underlying motivations for the introduction of compulsory citizenship education was to provide more uniform coverage of citizenship across schools in England. Nevertheless, challenges remain apparent in the quest for a common citizenship. In particular, Faulks (2006) argues that the government's policy focus on the diversification of school types and the inequalities inherent in the process of secondary school choice means that students are not necessarily receiving the 'common' approach to citizenship that the Crick Report advocated. Faith schools are especially problematic, as students are likely to be taught citizenship from one particular stance rather than having the opportunity to explore broader perspectives (Leighton, 2004; Faulks, 2006). Moreover, private schools are not expected to comply with the Citizenship Order (Faulks, 2006). Heater (2001) also shares such concerns, although he takes a more historical approach suggesting that past divisions in the education system, for example between private and state schools, and between grammar and secondary modern schools, reinforced class divisions and the uneven nature of education provision. The direction of dominant policies therefore do little to promote an inclusive and common approach to citizenship education.

Young people involved in the Children and Young People's Unit's consultation (CYPU, 2002) were concerned that the benefits of citizenship education would not be consistent in different schools. Despite the aspiration for a common approach to citizenship, context at the level of the individual school remains significant to the depth and quality of citizenship education received by students. Ireland *et al.* (2006a), in their longitudinal study of citizenship education, have devised a typology of approaches ranging from the most advanced schools that have developed citizenship in the curriculum, the school and wider community, to those schools that have a very limited approach. Furthermore, Clemitshaw and Calvert (2005) argue that the development of citizenship education is susceptible to different contexts within schools, citing the restructuring of staff and long-term illness of citizenship coordinators as factors which may affect the success of the subject. Individual schools and teachers may also adopt different perspectives on citizenship (Morrell, 1991), and the extent to which teachers are able to participate in decision-making within a school has obvious implications for teenagers' opportunities to contribute. In these terms, students' learning experiences still appear to vary widely.

Teachers' experiences

Whilst there is evidence to suggest that many teachers welcomed the introduction of compulsory citizenship education, the implementation of the subject has not gone without controversy. Drives towards assessing schools and young people through examination have to some degree resulted in the relegation of non-examined subjects such as citizenship (Heater, 2001; Leighton, 2004). Those teachers specializing in citizenship may, therefore, feel undervalued as non-examined subjects are often given low priority (Clemitshaw and Calvert, 2005; Crace, 2005).

The flexible approach schools can take to delivering the subject has led to confusion amongst teaching staff, many of whom have not received adequate training (Faulks, 2006). If schools are confused and unsure about the curriculum then this will have inevitable implications for the way young people view the subject. Crace (2005) argues that the government has not invested enough funding in the subject which would enable, for example, more specialist teachers to be trained. There is evidence to suggest that since the implementation of compulsory citizenship education there has been an increase in the number of teachers receiving training in the subject, although recent data also confirm that many still have not received any training (Crow, 2004; Leighton, 2004; Ireland *et al.*, 2006a). As a result many teachers also felt they needed more support. A lack of training and support undoubtedly leads to stress and anxiety amongst teachers and raises questions about the quality of citizenship education provision in different schools. Furthermore, the citizenship coordinators in Clemitshaw and Calvert's (2005) research stated that their role was an extra responsibility, which for many had not been accompanied by a salary increase.

Finally, in terms of fears regarding political indoctrination, the Crick Report attempts to allay parental concerns by stating that teachers are trained to be objective, impartial and balanced (QCA, 1998; Flew, 2000). It is, of course, unlikely that teachers can be truly objective. An analysis of teachers' attitudes towards engaging students with controversial issues conducted by Oulton *et al.* (2004) suggested that a lack of training had been detrimental to teachers' confidence. Fears over indoctrination also do not afford teenagers with political agency to question and challenge the views of their teachers. Moreover, whilst fears about indoctrination from individual teachers and schools have been of concern, little debate has centred upon the values promoted in state-based education, for example New Labour's focus on citizenship is undoubtedly concerned with fostering a particular kind of compliant citizen (see also Gordon *et al.*, 2000; Osler and Starkey, 2005b). Such values, Leighton (2004) argues, represent those of the 'chattering classes'.[8]

Teenagers' preliminary reactions

But what of teenagers' own attitudes towards the transition to compulsory citizenship education? Here I draw on teenagers' opinions and understandings of the citizenship curriculum both prior to and five months after the commencement of statutory citizenship education in order to ascertain the extent to which they were engaged in the subject. In this, I draw on survey, discussion and diary material from my research. The case study school chose to implement distinct citizenship lessons and in the view of the Office for Standards in Education (OFSTED) has done so successfully. The provision of education within the school is 'satisfactory' with GCSE results currently below the national average. The quality of provision of citizenship education, however, was graded as 'good' and was praised for strong leadership and excellent planning. The implementation of the subject through the 'pupil passport', where teenagers record their participation and responsibilities both inside and outside of school, was also highly regarded. My own observation in classes was that:

> Tutor time lasts for 35 minutes on a Friday morning, and most weeks citizenship is studied. They have recently all been given folders to keep

all their citizenship work in and, so far, they have mainly been looking at legal issues and laws. The form tutor had laid out their folders so I could take a look at them and several students seemed quite proud of them.

(Observations from Citizenship Class, 24th January 2003)

The school was seen to provide teenagers with a sound understanding of democracy, the rationale for adopting rules, and trust. In addition to weekly lessons the school also holds a biannual 'World Awareness Day' and a yearly 'Crime and Punishment Day'. Two of the teenagers in my study, Kitty Sandoral and Gumdrop, discussed the World Awareness Day:

KITTY SANDORAL: We're having this big day when all these ...
GUMDROP: Oh yeah well ... we're having World Awareness Day ... World Awareness Day that's something to do with citizens.

(Group discussion, 2nd July 2002)

Just before the transition to statutory citizenship lessons 425 teenagers aged 13–16 responded to a questionnaire survey. Just over half (53 per cent) of those surveyed were aware they had already been learning citizenship, although participation in this research may also have increased awareness to some extent. Similarly, none of the participants (aged 16–22) in Lister *et al.*'s (2001) study conducted prior to the introduction of compulsory citizenship education recalled having had any lessons explicitly on citizenship. Respondents in my own research were also asked to outline the citizenship-related topics which they recalled learning from a list of human rights, the government, voting, volunteering and community participation. Just under half (49 per cent) recalled learning about human rights, whilst around one-third remembered learning the other topics. Human rights (24 per cent) was deemed the most useful topic to learn, whilst volunteering was regarded as the least useful (13 per cent). In later discussions participants studied '*Citizenship: The National Curriculum for England – Key Stages 3–4 guide*' (QCA, 2000) in order to assess for themselves the extent to which they felt they would be engaged with the subject matter. Overwhelmingly, they deemed human and legal rights to have the potential to be the most interesting and useful aspects of citizenship education. The appeal of these subject areas highlighted participants' interests in local and global issues, as well as reflecting important transitionary changes in teenagers' lives. Nikki, for example, questioned the rationale underlying age-specific legislation:

Legal rights would probably be quite interesting because I'd like to know why we're not allowed to do it ... but adults are.

(Group discussion, 2nd July 2002)

At the same time human and legal rights were viewed as possessing future value. Bob told me that he felt that learning about legal rights would be helpful for adult life:

SUSIE: And I just wondered what ... if there are any subjects there you thought would be interesting or useful for you?
BOB: Um ... legal rights.
SUSIE: Yeah. Why do you think that might be useful?
BOB: Cos it's like good to know the umm ... law and everything cos it could like help you when you're older.

(Individual interview, 4th July 2002)

During the period of transition to compulsory citizenship lessons, relevancy was vital to teenagers' attitudes to the new curriculum. The popularity of human and legal rights relates very much to teenagers' understandings of their changing place within society as they approach key legal landmarks as citizens. Nevertheless, whilst participants were able to select potential areas of interest, the forthcoming curriculum was in general viewed with some disinterest. Just over half of those involved in in-depth elements of this research stated that they would not choose to study citizenship if it was an option. Gumdrop and Kitty Sandoral believe that it is not necessary to be taught citizenship at school because much of the subject can be learnt outside school:

SUSIE: If it was an option would you pick it?
GUMDROP/KITTY SANDORAL: Probably not! (Laughs)
SUSIE: Why not?
GUMDROP: Cos I think there's some things that are more important. Cos like there's stuff that you learn in lessons which you can only really learn at school. Stuff like this you could probably learn from other stuff like media and newspapers. That kind of thing.

(Group discussion, 2nd July 2002)

Only 23 per cent (n = 25) felt they would choose to study citizenship. Kendal and Tommey once again drew upon the notion of relevancy whilst deciding the worth of the subject:

SUSIE: If you had a choice over whether you picked it or not, do you think it would be a subject you would choose?
KENDAL: It depends really.
TOMMEY: It depends on what the other ones ... what the other options would be.
SUSIE: Yeah.

KENDAL: Yeah I dunno ... think about in later life what you were going to do ...
SUSIE: Yeah.
TOMMEY: Yeah.
KENDAL: Whether it's relevant.
TOMMEY: Yeah.

(Group discussion, 4th July 2002)

Furthermore, during the final few months before compulsory citizenship education was introduced, teenagers questioned the relevancy of the subject and whether citizenship had a place within an already packed curriculum:

> Why encourage people to do things that they don't want to do! There are not many people who want to something like a citizenship course. Just leave the kids alone, let them do what they want!
> (iwight web forum, Richard, 12th February 2003)

Before embarking upon citizenship education, participants' greatest concern was the relevance of the subject to their present lives. If their present lives are undervalued, this has the potential to affect teenagers' feelings of belonging and worth within society.

In January 2003 a second questionnaire was completed by 172 teenagers in year 10. It was designed to chart teenagers' views and reactions five months after the introduction of compulsory citizenship education. During the time that participants had been taking citizenship lessons they recalled having studied a variety of subjects including alcohol, drugs, smoking and solvent abuse; crime and law; sex education; the government; rights; and friendships. These recollections matched the actual syllabus participants had been studying, which demonstrates a heightened awareness of citizenship since the introduction of dedicated lessons. To some extent this may be a reflection of the presence of this research project within the school, although this would only account for heightened awareness amongst a small number of students.

In the second survey, many participants (58 per cent) stated that they were not enjoying citizenship lessons. There was no statistical relationship between participants' interest in citizenship education and their engagement with school more generally. Furthermore, there was no statistical difference between girls' and boys' engagement with the subject. A small minority (9 per cent) stated that they enjoyed everything relating to citizenship education. In terms of non-topic-based enjoyment factors, several respondents found citizenship lessons both informative and relevant:

> The topics are informative.
> (Male, aged 15)

They're good for our age because we're starting to do these things.

(Male, age unknown)

We cover issues that are relevant to everyday life.

(Male, aged 15)

A small proportion (6 per cent) of respondents also enjoyed voicing and discussing their opinions, whilst a small number (4 per cent) enjoyed working together as a class:

We always discuss the subject thoroughly making sure everyone understands.

(Unknown respondent)

The survey also asked respondents to 'send a message to the Prime Minister' in relation to their views on citizenship education. In total 8 per cent responded with positive comments on the introduction of the subject:

We should have more lessons.

(Female, aged 15)

It is a good idea and should be kept for future pupils.

(Male, aged 14)

It is very interesting and helpful to know what life will be like when you come out of school.

(Male, aged 14)

I think it is a good idea but there's a lot of room for improvement.

(Female, aged 15)

Teenagers who enjoyed their current citizenship classes were able to identify some kind of relevancy to their lives. This was principally in relation to the transition from childhood to adulthood. For those who were not enjoying citizenship lessons, the most common reason related to boredom (49 per cent). Several (12 per cent) stated that they had already studied the subject matter. More informal discussions highlighted relevancy as a key factor in teenagers' engagement with the subject:

Before the class started I spoke to one girl, who I had done a lot of work with before, and one boy, who had previously chosen not to be involved. They were quite happy to talk about their experiences although they were not all that positive. On the whole they found the subject boring. They felt that they either knew the subject matter before or that it was not relevant to them now. I asked them to compare citizenship to other lessons at school, and Lee felt that he preferred working in other lessons, although both he and Janna noted they had done a lot of work since the beginning of term.

(Observations from Citizenship Class, 24th January 2003)

Another important element was the delivery of such lessons. Several criticized the format of the lesson, complaining that they always had to fill in sheets or copy down notes:

> It's so boring because you only listen. You don't interact and learn anything you haven't already.
>
> (Female, aged 14)

> It is not interesting and the lessons are all of the same format.
>
> (Female, aged 14)

A minority of respondents did not enjoy citizenship lessons for several other reasons including disruptive behaviour by other members of the class, and a lack of time to cover topics sufficiently. Again, when asked to 'send a message to the Prime Minister' regarding citizenship education, a significant proportion of responses (30 per cent) were either negative or suggested areas for improvement:

> Don't bother, no-one pays attention.
>
> (Female, aged 14)

> We need to learn about real issues like war, violence.
>
> (Female, aged 14)

> Pupils should not be forced into doing it as a GCSE course.
>
> (Female, aged 15)

> That it is a waste of time and we shouldn't do it.
>
> (Male, aged 15)

A further 14 per cent utilized this part of the survey as a platform for airing other political views, using the research to create their own space of citizenship:

> We want peace.
>
> (Male, aged 14)

Ban fox hunting.

(Female, aged 14)

Screw citizenship, why don't you give us a reason for going to war?

(Male, aged 14)

Several respondents, therefore, reconstructed the questionnaire into their own space of citizenship to voice their opinions on a number of local and global issues. This indicates an absence of alternative platforms, which was indeed reinforced by several participants involved in interviews and diaries who thanked me for listening to their opinions, an opportunity most had never had before either within school or the wider community.

Since the transition to compulsory citizenship education, OFSTED has conducted a small-scale evaluation of the implementation of the subject. Having inspected twenty-five schools, OFSTED concluded that, whilst examples of good practice existed, progress in over half of the schools was unsatisfactory. There was a general lack of understanding of what was meant by citizenship and what the curriculum should encompass (Kerr *et al.*, 2003; OFSTED, 2003). As chapter 2 outlined, the definition of citizenship is highly complex and open to much interpretation. In the second questionnaire I asked respondents to outline their own understandings of 'citizenship'. For 19 per cent of those surveyed, citizenship did not mean anything, whilst a further 34 per cent did not respond to the question. In addition 6 per cent defined it just as a (sometimes boring) lesson:

A lesson which we have at school.

(Male, aged 14)

These respondents did not appear to associate citizenship with any areas of their life beyond the classroom. Several participants (16 per cent), however, defined citizenship as being a good or better citizen, as this respondent suggests:

Training to be good citizens.

(Unknown respondent)

For some this related to being a member of their country or more globally, whilst 8 per cent equated the notion to ideas of community and taking part in society:

How to be a good member of the community.

(Female, aged 14)

Rights and laws of people in the community.

(Female, aged 14)

It is apparent from such responses that citizenship is defined at a number of different levels, from local spaces to the wider global community. In the main, respondents reflected the more cosmopolitan notion of citizenship, outlined by McGrew (2000), which spans both local and global spheres but has little connection to the nation-state. Teenagers' perceptions (gathered in 2002 and 2003) paint a negative picture of contemporary citizenship education. Unfortunately this negativity also runs through other more recent quantitative studies. A survey commissioned by OFSTED found that 10 per cent of secondary school students still were not aware of citizenship classes (Crace, 2005). On a more positive note, research conducted by 'Community Service Volunteers' in 2004 found that a small, but significant number of students felt that learning citizenship fostered a greater sense of respect and tolerance for others (Crace, 2004). Schools deemed to be particularly successful are those in which citizenship is engrained in all aspects of school life. Despite this, coverage remains inconsistent (Crace, 2004).

The National Foundation for Educational Research (NfER) is currently conducting a nine-year longitudinal study exploring the implementation of citizenship education in England (Ireland and Kerr, 2004; Cleaver *et al.*, 2005; Ireland *et al.*, 2006a; 2006b). The research is charting the progress of over 10,000 students via survey as well as more in-depth case study work, in order to explore the short- and long-term implications of citizenship on young people's knowledge and skills. To date, findings from the research suggest that students have become progressively more aware that they are studying citizenship, and that on the whole citizenship has become more consolidated since 2002. More schools now teach citizenship as a discrete lesson, and include elements in extra-curricula activities. Many teachers are also more positive and confident about the likely effects of the subject, although confidence levels amongst teachers remain relatively low. In 2006 participants considered 'belonging', 'having a say' and 'opportunities for participation' as important aspects of citizenship. The 2006 report on NfER's longitudinal study focused upon active citizenship and forging links between citizenship education and other areas of policy concerned with civic renewal and participation, for example, through the government's civic renewal unit, and policy initiatives such as the *Youth Matters* Green Paper and the *Every Child Matters* programme, which promote participation and community involvement. More schools are now forging links with their communities, and schools themselves are being recognized as important communities for young people. The 'active' elements of citizenship were regarded by many schools as the hardest to implement, and school was often the only arena that students were afforded to practise citizenship. Whilst this longitudinal study reinforces the need to provide more opportunities for participation, there is little emphasis on how the curriculum could be strengthened by drawing upon teenagers' own experiences.

At present, citizenship education appears to have some way to go before the majority of teenagers are fully engaged with the subject matter. The key factors in the effectiveness of the curriculum lie with both relating the subject to teenagers' everyday lives (as well as their futures), in addition to broadening the definition of citizenship (education).

Recognizing alternative ways of learning citizenship

In charting the development of compulsory citizenship education in English secondary schools, as well as some of the conceptual and practical difficulties in fostering an effective curriculum, it has become apparent that there are several fundamental problems in the way citizenship has been conceived of in this policy initiative. Whilst in its current guise the curriculum seeks to tackle concerns regarding apathy and anti-social behaviour it fails to recognize both alternative and more holistic understandings of citizenship, which in many ways are more inclusive, and perhaps relevant to many teenagers' lives. A sustained focus on developing future, responsible, *compliant* citizens is also in danger of fuelling mistrust in formal politics. Moreover, on a practical level as Clemitshaw and Calvert argue:

> despite the best intentions and hard work of citizenship coordinators, the implementation of the citizenship curriculum is proving to be slow, uneven and uncertain.
>
> (2005: 35)

In essence, the implementation of citizenship has, in practice, been much more complex than was perceived during policy formation. Nevertheless, there are positive examples of schools developing effective practices where citizenship and democratic principles are at the heart of the school ethos.

A growing body of research suggests that for effective citizenship education children and young teenagers should be afforded opportunities to practise citizenship (see, for example, Hine *et al.*, 2004). As the proceeding chapters highlight, providing opportunities for experiencing and practising citizenship are important and valuable. At the same time pursuing this line of enquiry also presupposes, to some degree, that teenagers are not already engaged in acts of citizenship. It is perhaps more fundamental to develop mechanisms which enable teenagers' own experiences, interests and involvement to be central and drawn upon within both schools and wider society. Indeed, Biesta and Lawy (2006) call for more research and policy emphasis which examines the ways in which young people learn citizenship, arguing that:

> They [young people] learn as much, and most possibly even more, from their participation in the family or leisure activities, from interaction

with their peers, from the media, from advertising and from their role as consumers – and they often learn different and even contradictory things ... All this suggests that the learning of democratic citizenship is situated within the lives of young people.

(2006: 73)

I have already explored the practice of citizenship more generally, pointing to the unconventional and often unrecognized acts of citizenship in which many teenagers engage within their schools. This serves as an important lesson for the way the curriculum could take a broader, more relevant, more inclusive and more cosmopolitan stance to citizenship. Such an approach is fundamental if policy-makers are to avoid increasing teenagers' disaffection with formal politics; the opposite of their intentions. The following chapters therefore examine teenagers' citizenship in a number of arenas both within school and within the wider community.

Chapter 4

Practising citizenship in school

Introducing teenagers' citizenship in school

The case study school experienced a number of upheavals when I attended as a pupil over a decade ago. The head teacher had left under difficult circumstances and, whilst several inspirational teachers remained, the school lacked morale for a number of years. Achievement was not high and some classes were chaotic places where little was learnt academically but a great deal was learnt about life. This was a story of struggle for education and several key teachers took part in these 'battles', motivating students to stand up to the challenges. Whilst a school council existed it did not, at the time, appear effective and I recall that on several occasions my friends and I arranged an appointment with the head teacher to discuss our concerns about the quality of teaching and to air our views directly. As this chapter will show, the school has changed and is exhibiting many examples of effective practice. What my recollections have sought to highlight, though, is that teenagers are not simply passive within school. Many challenge the status quo often in unconventional and perhaps controversial ways. Nevertheless, young teenagers in compulsory education spend a substantial proportion of their lives under the authority of schools, but often have little opportunity to formally voice their opinions in a way that will bring about meaningful change (James *et al.*, 1998; Edwards, 2002; Thomas and Hocking, 2003). As Gordon *et al.* argue:

> The search for autonomy and independence is important to school students, who often talk about school in terms of conflicts between the necessity for 'discipline' and their own need for decision making.
>
> (2000: 14)

Continuing with the theme of citizenship in school this chapter explores teenagers' experiences of participation in decision-making. In light of the introduction of compulsory citizenship education, schools are also influential in the development of teenagers' political understandings and active citizenship. The overriding aim of this chapter is to reflect upon teenagers' understandings and experiences of citizenship within different aspects of everyday life at school. It draws attention to both the more formal aspects of citizenship in school such as the school council, as well as the informal school (see Gordon *et al.*, 2000). I begin by exploring citizenship as praxis within the classroom, particularly in relation to the teaching methods favoured by participants and the degree to which teenagers were engaged with citizenship as a subject. I also draw attention to the importance of subject relevancy in teenagers' present lives. For example, when deficit models of childhood and citizenship are disregarded in the classroom, this has a positive impact upon engagement with the subject. When teenagers felt that they were treated like adults or perhaps as equals, and where they were afforded the opportunity actively to make decisions over their learning, they were more likely to be engaged in citizenship education. The second section of this chapter examines participants' experiences of being listened to at school, informally by teaching staff and more formally through mechanisms such as the school council. Finally, less apparent forms of citizenship will be illustrated through the exploration of active citizenship during teenagers' 'free time' at school. Such spaces are important spheres for social and political interaction, as well as for the formation of social capital (Armstrong-Esther and Goodwin, 2003).

Practising citizenship in the classroom

Authors such as Hahn (1999) have drawn attention to the notion of the democratic classroom, derived from John Dewey's progressive work on democratic education (Dewey, 1916; see also Osler and Starkey, 2005b). The democratic classroom effectively promotes citizenship through the practice of democracy in school. Here I explore teenagers' experiences of citizenship as praxis within the classroom by highlighting participants' criticisms and preferences for the way in which citizenship is presented. Issues of subject relevancy are also discussed in order to emphasize the difficulties inherent in promoting citizenship education, which focuses on creating *future* responsible citizens.

Participatory learning methods

Much of contemporary citizenship education literature is bound to the notion of *active* citizenship (QCA, 1998; Chisholm, 2001). It would seem somewhat paradoxical, therefore, that in mainstream schooling children and teenagers have little opportunity to voice their opinions over *their* learning. Creating space within the curriculum for participatory learning is often challenging (Christensen *et al.*, 2000). Nevertheless, Griffith (1998) highlights that participatory education should be an essential element of citizenship. To explore the extent to which citizenship can be fostered within the classroom, this section examines teenagers' opinions on effective methods of teaching citizenship. Most participants preferred to be taught using a multi-method approach. The single most popular method was, however, the internet (mentioned by 52 per cent of respondents):

> I like using the internet and watching videos and the teaching is good too.
>
> (Unknown respondent)

This was followed by the use of videos/DVDs (mentioned by 47 per cent of respondents) and being taught by a teacher (mentioned by 37 per cent):

> I like the teacher because they can express their own way of learning and teaching.
>
> (Female, aged 14)

A small number of respondents viewed the use of textbooks (5 per cent) and group work (3 per cent) as popular methods. Several teenagers cited practical participation as a favourable teaching method. In one citizenship class, for example, teenagers learnt practical lessons about alcohol:

> I enjoyed the lesson on alcohol because we measured out the different units.
>
> (Male, aged 14)

The prevalence of traditional teaching methods appears to be relatively widespread. In NfER's longitudinal research the teaching methods employed by schools in the study in 2004 also remained predominantly didactic rather than participatory, although students did feel there was some room for discussion. By 2006 there had been a small increase in the use of less conventional teaching methods including the internet. Home literacy was also regarded as important in the development of political literacy and involvement (Cleaver et al., 2005; Ireland et al., 2006a; 2006b).

The most productive lessons were viewed by OFSTED as those which allowed participation in discussion. This view was echoed by many students:

> Talking with other class members helps us learn other information.
>
> (Female, aged 14)

Space to express beliefs and opinions in class discussions was valued by several teenagers (Weller, 2003). Drawing upon experiences in a science lesson, Nikki and Funda highlighted conflicts between teachers and pupils over preferred methods of learning:

NIKKI: ... and I told my teacher that I wanted to do that the other day and she turned around and shouted at me saying that we have to do what she wants to do because it's work and we have to get it done but we're not allowed to have fun like all the other classes.

FUNDA: Our teacher he ... cos we only have him for one lesson a week he actually sits there and says 'what do you want to do next lesson as long as it's scientific' ...

SUSIE: Oh.

FUNDA: ... so we get to choose what we do and he'll make it scientific for us

SUSIE: Do you think you learn more doing it that way?

FUNDA: Yeah. It's more fun. It sits in your head more as well.

NIKKI: Cos when you're bored in a lesson ...

FUNDA: It goes in one ear ...

NIKKI: ... you don't pay as much attention. Yeah it just goes in one ear and out the other. But if you're enjoying it you remember it.

(Group discussion, 2nd July 2002)

Nikki and Funda emphasize not only the different learning experiences that teenagers encounter but, importantly, the positive outcomes that participation in decision-making over learning can have (Weller, 2003). A study conducted in the USA revealed that the discussion of, and participation in, political issues was far more effective than civics education (Owen, 1996), as one questionnaire respondent reinforced:

I dislike the subject immensely as we are not allowed to discuss any of our own views ... we simply copy laws from a text book.

(Male, aged 14)

OFSTED praised the case study school in this research for inviting visitors to speak at citizenship lessons, especially as teenagers were given the responsibility to collect visitors from the reception when they arrived. Visitors do, however, need to possess suitable communication skills and to allow for discussion in their presentations. During my observation of one citizenship lesson, a visiting speaker purveyed some poignant messages to the class. She did so, however, in an authoritative, 'teacher-like' manner, ordering one teenager to 'stop chewing'. There was, in this session, some discussion although this was often in the form of the visitor asking the class questions rather than more open dialogue:

The lesson that day involved a talk from a representative from the [organisation], a drop-in advice centre/telephone helpline for young people. I sat on a table at the back of the class. The speaker talked of issues that are both relevant to young people now and in the future. After a while she introduced ideas for discussion through worksheets and hung these on a washing line. They covered issues of exclusion including 'loneliness', 'not fitting in' and 'bullying'. The class reacted quickly with answers, although there were varying degrees of participation in the class – this is probably usual within any class. One group of boys looked particularly bored.

(Observations from Citizenship Class, 24th January 2003)

The teaching methods chosen to deliver citizenship education are highly significant to the 'success' of the subject. Teenagers in this research favoured participatory methods, which enable them to make active contributions as citizens in school.

Subject relevancy

Prior to the commencement of statutory citizenship classes participants were asked, through the first questionnaire and discussions, whether they felt learning such material would be of use to them now, as teenagers, or in the future. Exploring this issue is fundamentally important to understanding the construction of teenagers as citizens. Overwhelmingly, with only one exception, all teenagers involved in the in-depth research stated that the subject matter would be of more use to them in the future. Such education was tied to adult activities which exclude teenagers of this age group. Janna, for example, suggests that her lack of interest in the subject is related to her exclusion from electoral politics:

SUSIE: Yeah. So do you think that learning about some of that kind of stuff would be useful for you now or more in the future?

JANNA: More in the future. Now cos I don't really care about voting or anything or who's the Prime Minister cos I don't really know much about it. As soon as I get to 18 where I can vote, I mean I'll start getting interested in it but it's just ... it's something I don't need to know at the moment so I'll probably be ...

SUSIE: So would you be interested if they like lowered the age of voting?

JANNA: Yeah, yeah I would if it was like 16 as soon as I've got to 16 I'll be interested and want to know what's going on in the parliament and stuff.

(Individual interview, 5th July 2002)

Teenagers' exclusion from mainstream, formal politics does not encourage engagement in citizenship as a curriculum subject. Despite this, Kitty Sandoral and Gumdrop highlight a contradiction. Whilst some teenagers appear not to be interested in the subject because they are not able to participate in formal participatory mechanisms, some do not feel confident or informed enough, for example, to vote:

SUSIE: Yeah, and do you think those topics will be useful for you now or can you see it being more use in the future?

GUMDROP: I think more use in the future.

KITTY SANDORAL: Well elections and voting and stuff like that will be useful in the future but some of it wouldn't really be ... you wouldn't really need it for us now. So mostly for the future.

SUSIE: Yeah. Would you like to vote now if you could?

GUMDROP: I think personally ... I think probably ... we don't know enough about parties that kind of thing to be able to vote now. You got to like ... if you had to vote now you'd have to learn more about what's going on.

SUSIE: Yeah.

KITTY SANDORAL: I feel that I'd be too influenced by other people and it would be difficult for people if they're not, like you said if they're not sure about things. They're just ... they're like 'oh well you should vote for my party' and then I'll vote for them or something like that.

(Group discussion, 2nd July 2002)

Janna, Gumdrop and Kitty Sandoral raise perhaps one of the greatest challenges facing teenagers' engagement with citizenship education. A fine balance is needed between teaching teenagers subject matter that is relevant to them as citizens-in-the-present whilst providing information and debate for their different roles as future citizens. To reinforce this point, many teenagers felt that certain aspects of citizenship education might be of use to their future roles as parents or to their careers. Funda highlights her interest in the role of law courts for her future career as a lawyer:

SUSIE: OK the topics that you're interested in are they useful for you now or more useful in the future?

FUNDA: I think ... I think that if we learn about certain things now we're gonna have more of an understanding in the future so I think it's both but it depends ... cos I know exactly what I'm going to do when I'm older when I leave school ...

SUSIE: Yeah.

FUNDA: ... and I have done since I was ten years old which I've had a very clear mind about that so I would be interested in like the role of law courts but I think the other stuff it's not gonna interest me at all.

(Group discussion, 2nd July 2002)

Many of the participants (aged 16–22) in Lister *et al.*'s (2001) study wanted citizenship education to help them develop skills which would be useful once they had left school. Participants in this study, however, were several years younger and had three more years of compulsory education ahead of them.

Participants' concerns that the subject should be relevant to both their present and future lives, to some extent, are reflected in the aims of the subject. The curriculum does promote the necessity to consider the needs of children and teenagers in terms of educational ability, gender and ethnicity as well as relating the subject to students' interests. The opening section of the curriculum guide for Key Stages 3 and 4 implicitly defines citizenship as a future status by suggesting that teenagers should merely be 'helpfully involved' in their schools and communities (QCA, 2000).

Five months after the introduction of compulsory citizenship education respondents were asked again when they felt the topics they were learning would be of use to them. This point was re-examined in order to assess differences between participants' perceptions of the subject prior to its compulsory implementation and their subsequent experiences. The majority (63 per cent) of participants felt that citizenship education would be useful to them both now and in the future. A minority (16 per cent) believed that citizenship education would be directly useful to them now as teenagers, whilst 21 per cent believed they would only be of value for the future. The majority (71 per cent) of participants felt that alcohol, drugs and smoking were the most useful topics to learn as teenagers. Sex education (19 per cent) and law and order (19 per cent) were also deemed to be useful to participants now:

> Sex education, drugs and drink so we know what we're getting ourselves into.
>
> (Male, aged 14)

> Law because I'm not from this country and didn't know what my rights were.
>
> (Female, aged 15)

A small number of respondents (7 per cent) believed that all the subject matter they had studied was of value to teenagers, highlighting the broader value of:

> Making your mind up about things.
>
> (Unknown respondent)

As Jenks (2001) suggests, the discourse of teenagers as 'becomings' is nowhere more fervently upheld than within the classroom as children and young people are constantly graded in terms of development. Although participants' emphasis on the future role of citizenship education would infer that the subject reinforces this discourse, thus rendering children and teenagers as 'human becomings' (see Cockburn, 1998; Prout, 2000), other findings from the survey did not reinforce this notion. Participants were asked how they felt they were treated within such lessons. Most (72 per cent) of those surveyed felt that they were treated either as young people or adults in citizenship classes, with only 12 per cent feeling that they were treated like children. Fundamentally, the status that participants were afforded in these terms shaped their interest in the subject. There was a statistical relationship (99 per cent level of significance) between how participants felt they were regarded by teachers and their level of interest in citizenship education (see table 1). All of those participants who felt treated like children during citizenship lessons did not like the subject. The more teachers treated participants as adults, the more likely they were to be interested in the lesson. This finding has significant implications for the effectiveness of the curriculum, as well as teenagers' broader societal status.

Table 1 Perceptions of status and enjoyment of citizenship education

| | | How do you feel you are treated when you are taught citizenship? (%) | | |
		As a child (n = 21)	As a young person (n = 87)	As an adult (n = 36)
Are you enjoying citizenship?	Yes	0	39	72
	No	100	61	28

n = 144

Davies *et al.* (1999) have drawn attention to the notion of the 'hidden curriculum' or the encounters within a school that are educational but not necessarily an explicit part of the curriculum. This 'hidden curriculum' may be applied to how teenagers are required to refer to teachers. In these terms the school ethos has important implications for both citizenship education and the status teenagers believe they are afforded. The participants in this research also suggested that the approach of individual teachers, as well as school ethos, significantly affected teenagers' engagement with citizenship.

Prior to the introduction of compulsory citizenship education respondents were asked if they felt learning about citizenship would encourage them to be interested in their communities. Participants were shown a list of citizenship-related topics (DfEE and QCA, 1999; QCA, 2000). From those who responded, only 31 per cent (n = 342) felt it would make them more interested. In later in-depth discussions there was a mixed response to this question, with just over half suggesting that learning citizenship in school would not impact upon their interest in community issues outside school, as for Janna:

SUSIE: Do you think that learning some of those subjects would be um ... make you be more interested in what goes on in your community? Will they help you?

JANNA: No, I don't think so. I wouldn't say that it would be one of my immediate reactions to 'Oh I want to learn something about my community. Let's learn human rights'. I wouldn't say that if you know what I mean.

(Individual interview, 5th July 2002)

Some respondents did not see how the lessons learnt in citizenship education could be practically applied to their everyday lives. Indeed, Davies *et al.* (1999) infer that there is often a cleavage between schools and their surrounding communities. The absence of links among schools and communities may contribute to the difficulty that some participants face in relating lessons learnt in citizenship to their own life-worlds. For those who believed citizenship education would have a tangible influence on their interest in community life, specific topic areas were highlighted as the most useful for engagement in local issues:

SUSIE: Do you think learning about some of those things would make you more interested in what goes on in your communities now?

KENDAL: Dunno.

TOMMEY: I think so cos you learn how it's sort of run and stuff.

SUSIE: Yeah.

TOMMEY: ... so you might be able to see the way you can help out and that ... sort of weaknesses and stuff you could help fix. Things like that.

KENDAL: Yeah like I just said again you'd know what was going on with the council and stuff ... all the people around ...

SUSIE: Yeah.

KENDAL: ... what they're doing with the money and stuff but cos ... I suspect certain towns get money, don't they? ... to spend on things and it would be good to know what they're doing with your money.

SUSIE: Yeah that's true.

MATT: It would be quite good to understand what's happening.

(Group discussion, 4th July 2002)

In the above discussion Kendal, Matt and Tommey outlined a number of 'real-life' scenarios relating to topics in the curriculum. In the second questionnaire just over one-third (36 per cent; n = 133) of those who had participated in a local project, campaign or voluntary work believed that the topics covered in citizenship had helped them with their project or campaign. Moreover, there was a statistical relationship (95 per cent level of significance) between whether participants were enjoying citizenship education and their involvement in a local campaign. Teenagers who had been involved in a local issue, campaign or project were more likely to be enjoying citizenship lessons (55 per cent). Equally, those respondents who had not participated in their communities were more likely to dislike such lessons (68 per cent). A pre-existing interest in the community, on whatever basis, appears to aid engagement in the citizenship curriculum. These participants may, therefore, bring their own sense of 'subject relevancy' to the classroom.

Eighteen respondents outlined the ways in which they felt citizenship lessons had aided their project or campaign. Some responses suggested that learning citizenship helped with practical issues:

> In law e.g. how we can campaign for a skate park in a proper way.
>
> (Male, aged 14)

This questionnaire respondent highlighted how citizenship lessons enabled him to make planning and campaigning decisions over new skate-park facilities. Here, citizenship education has practical outcomes for specific projects. Lessons in citizenship were also valuable in developing wider skills which could be applied to local participation:

> I think it makes you more sensible.
>
> (Female, aged 14)

> Responsibility.
>
> (Male, aged 14)

> They've taught you about the outside world.
>
> (Male, aged 14)

> They make me more aware.
>
> (Female, aged 15)

The skills these participants described are central to the philosophy of the citizenship curriculum. Moreover, from the entire target population for the survey just over one-third (36 per cent) believed that taking part in citizenship lessons had made them think about participating in a campaign, community project or to volunteer in the future. It should perhaps be acknowledged that respondents may have been relaying the rhetoric of citizenship. Nevertheless, as I will detail in chapter 5, several participants were able to demonstrate their own practical engagements with citizenship. The approach and delivery of citizenship education is fundamentally important to teenagers' understandings of democracy and citizenship and is likely to affect their future participation and inclusion. The enhanced engagement in citizenship education of teenagers who are or have been actively involved in their communities is highly significant. In conjunction with formal lessons, the ethos and spaces of citizenship within the wider school are also essential to the engagement of teenagers. As Alderson (2000b) suggests, children and young people become democratic citizens through praxis. I now explore participants' experiences of being heard at school.

Being heard at school

Citizenship education is only likely to appear relevant to teenagers if it is reinforced with opportunities to actually practise citizenship within school (Lister *et al.*, 2001). A participatory ethos within a school, therefore, is fundamental to an effective citizenship curriculum. Other studies have cited examples of good practice in which student participation is an integral part of a school's ethos, even involving very young children. Such an approach can have positive effects upon not only pupil empowerment but also achievement (Moggach, 2006). Indeed, the curriculum guidelines suggest that members of the school should have the opportunity to be 'helpfully involved' (QCA, 2000). The extent to which teenagers feel able to act as citizens and have their opinions respected has the potential to shape their engagement with citizenship education and the wider community. So what are teenagers' experiences of active citizenship within school in relation to the extent to which they feel their voices are listened to on an everyday basis by staff, and more formally through the school council?

Informal participation

Wyness (1999) suggests that, despite recent education reform which places emphasis upon 'choice', children have less opportunity for participation since the passing of the 1986 Education Act. This legislation, which Wyness believes does not adhere to the UNCRC, withdrew children's status on school governing bodies. As outlined in chapter 1, the UNCRC states that children and young people have the right to be consulted over matters which impact upon their lives (Muscroft, 1999; Alderson, 2000b). This section examines the extent to which participants felt their opinions were listened to by teaching staff in everyday settings. Outside of structures such as the school council some teenagers felt that, in general, teachers listened to their opinions and concerns, as Janna stresses:

> It's a good ... good school. It's um ... It does listen to young people even though most people wouldn't think it does, but it does do it.
>
> (Individual interview, 5th July 2002)

For several participants, the school set a better example of good participatory practice than they had previously experienced:

CHLOE: But um ... like sometimes um ... people go to the head of year and like say stuff and sometimes it doesn't um ... get taken into consideration but most of the time if you do like complain about something it will get um ... um ... something done about it.

KATIE: Yeah. But at our other school nothing was really done. If you like complained about the toilets or something ... something that needs to be done they wouldn't do it ... but here it's better.

(Group discussion, 3rd July 2002)

The opportunity to consult with teachers is, therefore, dependent upon the ethos of individual schools. One limitation of my study is that participatory practices in different schools could not be evaluated. Nevertheless, participants were able to draw upon their own diverse experiences to illustrate differences between schools.[9] Moreover, within a relatively large secondary school the opportunities available for voicing opinions varied between different individuals. Some felt that teachers had little time to take on board everyone's point of view, as Rammstein Nut notes:

Our teachers try to listen to our views on certain things but sometimes they just have too many people to deal with.

(Extract from Rammstein Nut's diary)

There were inevitable instances where teenagers believed that individual teachers were not good at listening to their views, as Bob highlights:

SUSIE: Do you feel listened to at school?

BOB: Umm ... most of the time. Like in [teacher] lesson ... (Pause) umm ... he like ... he doesn't listen to you ... if you ask a question he tells you to put your hand up and when you put your hand up he tells you to put your hand down and stuff, and then he just chucks you out even if you haven't done anything and that's just not funny cos you have to stand outside.

(Individual interview, 4th July 2002)

This also reflects findings from Lister *et al.*'s study which suggested that students had varying opportunities to effect change more informally through consultation with teaching staff, and suggested that particular teachers were more likely to listen to some students over others (Lister *et al.*, 2001). Funda and Nikki further this point by suggesting that some teachers had favourite students whose opinions were more likely to be acknowledged:

FUNDA: I've got favourite teachers ...

NIKKI: Yeah so have I.

FUNDA: They listen to you. Miss [Teacher] does. She's definitely the best teacher but some of the teachers ...

NIKKI: If they don't like you from the beginning of the year they won't like you at the end ...

FUNDA: Yeah.

NIKKI: ... they don't change their opinion of you. They just keep it.

FUNDA: And I don't think that's fair. They all say ... the teachers think they're always right and if you try and say 'no' and give your opinion it's like 'don't talk back to me ... blah, blah, blah'. You just get shouted [at] when you don't exactly set off to talk back to them you try and say something.

NIKKI: Yeah. They like say you should treat teachers how you want to be treated but they don't treat you the same no matter how you treat them.

FUNDA: It needs to work both ways.

(Group discussion, 2nd July 2002)

Funda and Nikki highlight the need for respect and egalitarianism in school to avoid undermining teenagers' status. They continue by suggesting that there is little room for free thinking and discussion within school. They also believed that as 'louder' teenagers, they were less likely to be listened to and instead felt they were seen in a derogatory light. Holland (2001) also found that greater credence was often given to the voices of 'sensible' children in the research scenario. Funda and Nikki believed that the listening ethos upheld by some teachers was not always put into practice. At the same time, Rammstein Nut felt that quiet teenagers who voice their opinions less explicitly are not necessarily less active citizens:

RAMMSTEIN NUT: Yeah ... um ... I don't really like to um ... make my opinion, you know, cos um ... I don't know ... I don't like talking out, you know ...

SUSIE: Yeah.

RAMMSTEIN NUT: ... go in front of the class and stuff like that but if it's on something ... I'm interested in history a lot at the moment with the war and I like to take my opinion in class, you know, give my views of it.

(Individual interview, 2nd July 2002)

On the whole, opinion was divided over whether teenagers felt listened to by teachers at school. This very much depended on individual experiences in different lessons. Participants in Hine *et al.*'s (2004) study advocated pro-social modelling, for example, teachers complying with the same school rules as students. The informal experiences of being heard are essential in creating environments within schools which both uphold the teachings of citizenship and encourage teenagers' active engagement. Without such an ethos schools could engender feelings of despondency amongst teenagers (Alderson, 2000b). This draws attention also to a more formal mechanism for the expression of teenagers' views within school – the school council.

The school council

Education on democracy can only be taught through praxis and not as an abstraction (Hart, 1992; Alderson, 2000c). Although some schools have young representatives on governing bodies (Edwards and Fogelman, 1991), many teenagers' experience of practising democracy is through a school council (Weller, 2003; Wyness, 2003). As Alderson states:

> School councils are a key practical and symbolic indicator of respect for children's rights.
>
> (2000b: 124)

Such a forum has the potential to provide teenagers with a stake in their school, often creating a more effective learning environment (McCulloch, 2000; Crick, 2002; James and James, 2004). Some schools have also discovered that developing active school councils can have a positive impact upon students' behaviour more generally (Alderson, 2000b).

In 1999 the National Society for the Prevention of Cruelty to Children (NSPCC) conducted a sample evaluation of schools in England and Wales to assess, in part, the role that school councils can play in providing children and young people with a stake in school decision-making (Baginsky and Hannam, 1999). They found that in the majority of schools, young people were able to contribute to the agenda of meetings. In just over half of the councils, however, some restrictions were placed upon the subjects discussed, for example, individual members of staff. In some cases school councils only explored trivial issues which, Davies et al. (1999) believe, have the potential to be more harmful than productive. Other schools provided opportunities for representatives to be involved in more substantial decision-making, for example, employing new members of staff (Baginsky and Hannam, 1999; OFSTED, 2003; Hudson, 2005), as well as acting as mediators and providing peer support (James and James, 2004). Overall, such councils were seen to be advantageous as they provided young people with a voice and helped to improve relations between staff and students. Limitations of time and resistance from teachers were outlined by staff as potential difficulties in developing effective school councils, whilst students felt that forging trusting relationships between staff and students was essential (Baginsky and Hannam, 1999).

In 2002 the International Association for the Evaluation of Educational Achievement (IEA) conducted the International Citizenship Education Study in twenty-eight countries. The research revealed that many of the 14-year-old respondents surveyed felt they had good opportunities to participate at school (Kerr et al., 2002). Either through formal or informal means, many participants believed they could bring about change, particularly when part of a group. Engagement in the school council, Kerr et al.

(2002) suggest, can have a significant effect upon both teenagers' engagement with citizenship education as well as their future political participation. Despite this, for many young people, the school council has little real impact upon their interest in citizenship education as participation is indirect and only achieved through their class representative (OFSTED, 2003).

Within the case study school there were mixed feelings about the effectiveness of the school council. Whilst ideologically it was deemed to be good practice, Janna, a class representative, had not been inspired to participate:

SUSIE: Are you involved in the school council?
JANNA: I am yeah. I don't go though (Laughs). I'm meant to go every Tuesday or something but I just forget. They don't put any reminders up or anything. Umm so ...
SUSIE: What were the meetings that you have been to been like?
JANNA: I've been to one. A whole year at school and I've only been to one council meeting! (Laughs). Not very good! Um ... (Laughs)...
(Individual interview, 5th July 2002)

Janna felt she needed more guidance and encouragement as class representative. She was not always aware when meetings were taking place as the council did not regularly meet on Tuesdays. Her own disengagement ultimately affected the engagement, and perceptions, of the school council's effectiveness by other teenagers (Weller, 2003). This echoes Kerr *et al.*'s (2002) observations that not all young people wish to participate in this format. Kerr *et al.* (2002), however, fail to acknowledge that what motivates individuals to participate can change rapidly and is often dependent on factors such as peer pressure, efficacy and the nature of subject matter discussed. A number of studies have also shown that school councils can be tokenistic and ineffective (Hine *et al.*, 2004), with several suggesting that teachers would do as they wished regardless of students' views (Lister *et al.*, 2001). Alderson's (2000b) comprehensive survey of school councils suggested that less than one-fifth of young people found the forum to be effective.

Several participants in this research believed the school council was effective. Many teenagers believed that it provided a much needed forum to voice their opinions in addition to raising awareness of their perspective(s) as teenagers. This is fundamentally important to the creation of engaging citizenship lessons. Teenagers are likely to become disengaged or disillusioned with citizenship as a subject if they do not experience real examples within school (Alderson, 2000b). Several participants also felt that within the context of wider decision-making, teenagers' views should be taken seriously. The school council, therefore, has the potential to bridge gaps and counter adultist assumptions that experiences of their own past youth gives them an insight into the lives of teenagers today. Many felt they were 'growing up' in a very different world, as Janna argued:

SUSIE: Do you think the school council is quite effective?
JANNA: Oh yeah, cos then [teacher] gets to hear our views on what we think is good for the school because as we know ...
SUSIE: Yeah.
JANNA: ... cos we're like part of it. It's hard for him to ... be in our shoes even though he has been, you know it's hard for him to like the same stuff we like. It's hard for him to imagine what it's like for us and stuff.
(Discussion with Janna, 5th July 2002)

Several participants cited examples of how the school council had brought about tangible benefits. Loki and Agnuz highlighted one such example:

LOKI: We did ask for some pool tables, didn't we?
AGNUZ: Oh yeah.
LOKI: We asked the teachers um ... the student council asked the teachers if we could have some pool tables er ... we got them.
(Group discussion, 3rd July 2002)

Not only does Loki cite a positive outcome of the school council but he makes reference to the school council being synonymous with the teenagers in the school, quite distinct from a collaboration between staff and students. Many of those involved in the in-depth elements of the research had not used the school council. Some simply had had no reason to raise an issue or request, whilst others were more sceptical of the school council's efficacy:

SUSIE: Do you use the school council or anything like that?
KIMBO: No I don't use the school council.
KAT: No.
KIMBO: No cos teachers never listen so.
(Group discussion, 4th July 2002)

A further reason for cynicism about the school council was that some felt other teenagers did not take its presence seriously, making what were deemed as 'silly' requests. As schools are so rigidly structured, children and young people are rarely consulted over the curriculum (Sibley, 1995; James et al., 1998; Prout, 2000). It is, therefore, hardly surprising that some doubt the effectiveness of the school council (Weller, 2003). Chloe suggests that this sometimes occurs when the class representative requests suggestions to take forward to the council:

If she does like the boys just mess around and stuff and put stupid stuff down ...

(Group discussion, 3rd July 2002)

As a result of these 'silly' requests some teenagers felt that teachers would not take other issues seriously:

People do ask for really stupid things. So they're not always sure whether you're being serious or something.

(Discussion with Gumdrop, 2nd July 2002)

Constructing meaningful spaces of citizenship within a school, therefore, is challenging. Indeed, different individuals or groups of teenagers have opposing ideas on what is legitimate to discuss in the school council. There was no evidence to suggest that those who made 'silly' requests were those more likely to feel excluded from participatory practices. It may be that these teenagers also declined to participate in this research. Nevertheless, the potential of the school council was broadly recognized. Kendal, Matt and Tommey also commented that the effectiveness of the school council relies not only on class representatives and teachers but with the participation of the whole school:

SUSIE: Would you like to have your opinion listened to more on stuff that goes on?

KENDAL: I would like to yeah.

TOMMEY: Yeah it would be better.

MATT: It would be better cos ... and what could be better ...

KENDAL: Cos like house captains and stuff go to the meetings. They don't really talk to the class about what's going on. It might be better if we all got involved in like what we could buy and stuff. I think the school could give us money to like buy stuff ... like it would be good if everybody had an opinion.

(Group discussion, 4th July 2002)

Malik (2002) calls for the (re)instatement of student governors, to work alongside school councils and to have greater influence over the running of the school. The practice of citizenship within school is subject to barriers and complexities ingrained in the education system, which relate to the construction of power relations between staff and students. Mechanisms such as school councils have done much to increase teenagers' stake within the school, but on an everyday basis teenagers' opportunities to shape their own experiences of citizenship and citizenship education are challenged. The school council is, however, only one way in which teenagers create spaces for themselves within school (Wyness, 2003), as I now discuss.

Citizenship in the informal school

Teenagers' use of time and space within school is heavily structured and controlled by adults. In the case study school one member of staff is 'on call', patrolling non-classroom areas for truants during lesson time. Jenks' (2001) exploration of embodiment highlights the temporal discipline of children's bodies within classroom spaces. He draws upon Durkheim and Foucault to suggest that time spent within the classroom is subject to control and constraint, and identifies the timetable as a metaphor for modernity in the way it regulates children's bodies in time and space. Such control is often lessened a little during break-times when more choice over use of space is available (Christensen *et al.*, 2000; Mayall, 2000). Time spent in school outside of the classroom would appear to equip teenagers with relative freedom. This section examines the micro-politics of citizenship within school, commencing by contextualising the spaces and activities participants engage in during their 'free time' at school. This is followed by discussions concerning the ways in which teenagers often overcome regulation and deal with conflict. I argue that these everyday negotiations of micro-politics are important learning experiences with regard to citizenship.

Politics in the playground

One element of the citizenship curriculum is political literacy (Lister *et al.*, 2001). Whilst this principally focuses upon more formal and often national institutions, the micro-politics of the playground arguably engage children and teenagers in smaller scale elements of democracy, such as learning about power relations, negotiating and mediating conflict, and participating in shaping spaces and relationships with peers and teaching staff. These micro-politics are of fundamental importance to the consideration of citizenship, for they reveal much about the political actions of and relationships between individuals and groups (see, for example, Gordon *et al.*, 2000). Students in English schools have longer break-times and correspondingly more time in the informal school than their counterparts in, for example, Finland (Gordon *et al.*, 2000). Exploring the places which teenagers value, claim and shape either within school or in the wider community provides an insight into the complex power relations manifested in those arenas. Within school, teenagers are not simply subject to control and regulation, but they exert agency, challenge power and carve out alternative niches particularly within the informal school (see also Gordon *et al.*, 2000). Teenagers' spatial and friendship allegiances provided a distinct geography of hanging out during 'free time' at school. As Holloway and Valentine (2000b) describe, teaching areas are often designated as 'out-of-bounds' during break-times. Except in bad weather, members of the school are expected to spend break and lunchtimes outside the school building but within the school boundaries, unless they go home for lunch. Kitty Sandoral highlighted the regularity of socializing in the same places:

> Anyway you get different people hang out in different places ...
> (Group discussion, 2nd July 2002)

Janna discussed the area in which she regularly hangs out:

SUSIE: So do you hang out in any particular place around school?
JANNA: Yeah you do. Yeah umm ... ours is kind of like the whole of the ... as you go round the main entrance ... ours is like the whole of that area ... the benches and the walls and the bars and the bike shed and stuff like that. That's where we mainly hang.
(Individual interview, 5th July 2002)

The geographies of hanging out at school are often determined by the structure of friendship groups and the preferred activities of those groups. Kendal, for example, spends much of his time taking part in sports with friends (see plate 1):

> At break and lunchtime I played basketball in the sports centre with my friends.
> (Extract from Kendal's diary)

Such places are, however, subject to change, especially through the progression of the school year. As new cohorts join and leave the school, spaces within the playground become (re)territorialized to suit the needs of new social groups, as Rammstein Nut detailed:

> If it's in school it's mainly up at the grass ... er ... the bank. It used to be the wall but now my friends have gone so there's more people that have taken it over.
> (Individual interview, 2nd July 2002)

The geographies of such micro-politics also change throughout the school year depending upon what activities are available. These variations are also determined by the season and weather, as Kitty Sandoral explained (see plate 2):

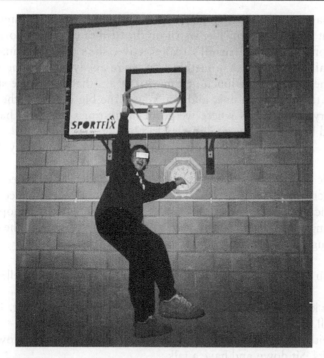

Plate 1 Hanging out in the basketball court, photographed by Kendal

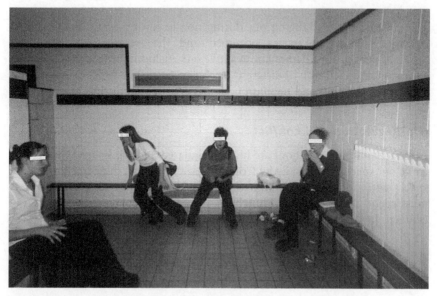

Plate 2 Hanging out in the changing rooms, photographed by Kitty Sandoral

... We hang out in the changing rooms more during the winter and stuff, but when it's sunny like we sit on the field or cos we're normally doing something cos [friend]'s really active, she's always doing like basketball or football or something, so we're always doing one thing or another at break or lunch ... Um ... that's ... that's the little sports hall cos there's a little one, and you've got the big one with the gym and everything. That's where we go in break-times and play basketball, and lunchtimes we go and play football or something.

(Group discussion, 2nd July 2002)

The rationale for the kinds of spaces chosen around the school reflects, for some teenagers, the desire to spend time away from adult surveillance. This may be particularly pertinent within a school setting where the panoptican of the teaching staff is ever present. Kaz, Kat and Kimbo discussed the areas that they hang out in to escape scrutiny:

SUSIE: Do you hang out in particular places around the school as well?
ALL: Yeah.
KAT: Do you know where the big bench is and the wall goes like that. That's where all of our friends sit and that.
KIMBO: We either go down the field or down the green room. Just down by the tracks. Sit down and have a talk.
SUSIE: Yeah.
KIMBO: So no teachers can bother us.

(Group discussion, 4th July 2002)

The geographies of hanging out during non-lesson time at school are distinctive. The actual spaces occupied and the (re)territorialization by different peer groups demonstrate active citizenship in practice through the exclusion and inclusion of different teenagers. Some teenagers can also challenge the restriction and regulation of spaces at school during break-times.

(De)Regulation and conflict

All spaces within the school are highly regulated and whilst many teenagers carve out specific places, away from the gaze of adults, their freedom to use spaces within the school is limited. As previously acknowledged, teenagers must spend their break and lunchtimes outside except when eating in the canteen. Janna does not agree with such regulation:

At break we all bundled inside cos it was very cold and windy but most of the teachers tell us to go outside! Which is really cruel.

(Extract from Janna's diary)

Learning spaces and leisure spaces appear to be delineated within the school. For those choosing not to eat in the school canteen, a prefabricated building has been created in the playground, set aside from the school:

> At lunchtime we went into the mobile cabin to have lunch because it is better than eating outside in the cold.
>
> (Extract from Chloe's diary)

Nevertheless, these regulations are challenged by some. Bob noted how he and his friend persistently challenge these rules, attempting to hang out within the school building, thereby redefining the intended and segregated learning/leisure spaces:

SUSIE: Is that like where you normally hang out at school?

BOB: No, normally I just run around inside the school building ... In school I just stay inside the school building and get told off all the time, at lunch and break cos ...

SUSIE: You're not allowed to stay in at lunch and break then?

BOB: Yeah. We don't ... me and my best friend, he like doesn't like it outside I just ... we just go wherever like ... he goes where I want and I go where he wants.

SUSIE: Oh that's nice.

BOB: Like we've basically been best friends since play school and umm ... whenever I'm not in he doesn't really hang out with anyone else. He just walks around on his own ...

SUSIE: Yeah.

BOB: Cos he doesn't really have many other friends except for me.

SUSIE: So do you get moved on a lot by the teachers then?

BOB: Yeah. Then we just walk off and ignore them most of the time.

SUSIE: What kind of places? Anywhere inside school or any ...?

BOB: Yeah, normally we come up the history, maths block or down the drama studio or hang out in the library and like ... umm ... they said that I was going to be suspended for ten days if I went in the library at lunchtime.

SUSIE: Why is that?

BOB: Because ... umm ... I got chucked out and kept going in there every day and asking if I was allowed back in there.

(Individual interview, 4th July 2002)

Rammstein Nut echoes Bob's experiences, highlighting the sometimes nomadic nature of hanging out especially when trying to challenge the spaces they can use:

> I try to stay indoors sometimes and we always get kicked out by teachers ... or we just move somewhere else around the school ...
>
> (Individual interview, 2nd July 2002)

Furthermore, certain spaces within the school building can offer some kind of immunity against having to go outside. One such space is the library, a much cited location for remaining indoors. As with Jenks' (2001) observations of children's re-regulation of their classroom activities, pretending to work whilst covertly writing notes to one another, the library, a seemingly work-related space, became an indoor place in which to socialize. Rammstein Nut, however, relates that simply hanging out near the library is often not seen as a legitimate reason for staying inside:

> Hung around near the library at school for a while until we got kicked out.
>
> (Extract from Rammstein Nut's diary)

The period between the end of break or lunch times and the start of lessons signifies a challenging time in teenagers' use of space within the school for, having left their 'free time' spaces, they enter more highly regulated space of the classroom. This control, Katie believed, is significantly linked to trust:

> When we are waiting to go into class at the end of lunch he [teacher] just locks the door and says: 'you can't go in because you all can't be trusted without a teacher'. That's more or less what he says. It gets on my nerves.
>
> (Extract from Katie's diary)

Some teenagers challenge teachers' authority by questioning their use of space in and around the school during break-times. Participants' challenges to regulation within school highlight a number of citizenship-related issues, including those of trust and respect in the teacher–pupil relationship and, moreover, teenagers' spatial autonomy, agency and decision-making abilities. One of the key elements of the citizenship curriculum, social and moral responsibility, focuses upon fostering responsible behaviour (Lister *et al.*, 2001) which implicitly suggests compliance with authority. It is again apparent that the definition of citizenship used in the curriculum does not provide space for conflict and struggle, which more 'alternative' understandings of citizenship value.

The politics of the playground are also shaped by conflicting interests between the teenagers themselves. As for Willis's (2001) examination of countercultural groups within schools, specific places were important signifiers of status within the school or within peer groups and were often determined by safety and/or identity (Weller, 2003). The 'smokers' or 'chimney boys', described by Loki below, hang out away from the adult gaze behind a tree in the playing field farthest from the school building. In doing so, the 'chimney boys' demonstrate their agency, opposing the structures and rules of the school. In detailing the activities of the 'chimney boys', Loki presents them as 'other'. Moreover, Loki and Agnuz opt to spend time in areas away from the smokers with whom they have come into conflict and by whom to some extent they feel threatened:

SUSIE: Do you usually go to the same places round school?
AGNUZ: Yeah.
LOKI: Yeah we've got our own little places. We ... we hang around the back of the school. We hang around on the grass. We go down to the other field. We play football and stuff like that. We just [ed] round the back ... and then you've got smokers' hedge down the bottom of the field. We don't go down there ... everybody just smokes. Um ... and then you've got the tree they smoke behind there. We don't go there ...
SUSIE: Is that the farthest bit from the school?
LOKI: Yeah the bit down there by the hedge ... They go down there and there's a tree at the front. They go behind there and they used to throw stuff at us when we used to play near there ... they used to throw mud.
(Group discussion, 3rd July 2002)

Here, Loki and Agnuz's example illustrates the power relations between one dominant and one resistant group of teenagers (see Sharp *et al.*, 2000), which ultimately led to Loki and Agnuz excluding themselves from an area of the school. Whilst Hey's (1997) ethnography illustrated conflicts amongst girls' friendship groups, this research did not highlight tensions based upon gender. Rather, conflict was often centred upon age (Tucker and Matthews, 2001), as Bob suggested:

SUSIE: How about in school, are there any places you don't feel comfortable in?
BOB: Sometimes I don't feel comfortable in the year 11 base [common room], um ... year 10 base because ... um ... there's a load of year 10s that don't like me for some reason.
(Individual interview, 4th July 2002)

Furthermore, Rammstein Nut also chose to hang out by the 'fatwall' primarily because she felt safe and comfortable there with her older friends:

RAMMSTEIN NUT: Oh yeah. We used to ... er um ... when my friends ... most of my friends are in the 11th year and they've all left and we used to hang out by this ... the wall near the bus shelter but they've all gone now so we ... I just sit with some of my 9th year friends and we sit up on the grass. It's like a little refuge thing ...

SUSIE: Yeah.

RAMMSTEIN NUT: ... cos with the 11th years I felt really safe and now I'm with the 9th years I just, you know, don't feel secure. With the 11th years they'd all protect me and that ... cos they were like my best friends. But they've all done their GCSEs now and left. Except for about two of them.

(Individual interview, 2nd July 2002)

Teenagers often reinforce adult gradations of age (Alderson, 2002; Mayall, 2002). Indeed, Corsaro (1997) notes that peer culture is both influenced by, and embedded in, broader adult cultures. This ultimately shapes who individuals construct as 'other'. Many of the participants interviewed in this research were amongst the youngest in the school and often noted conflicts with older children. Furthermore, 'sameness' and 'difference' (see Tucker, 2003) was often centred upon identity group cultures. I look at this issue further in chapter 5.

Teenagers challenge one another's hegemony in particular places of 'hanging out'. The political geographies of the playground are, therefore, highly dynamic and subject to constant change as peer groups reorganize and teenagers become more established within the school. Teenagers learn much about citizenship through their everyday encounters at school. Examining the micro-politics of such experiences highlights hidden geographies of citizenship, illustrating young teenagers' active roles in making decisions over spaces of inclusion and exclusion (Weller, 2003). Schools are fundamentally influential in fostering social connections, and, therefore, are implicated in shaping identity and social, economic and political life for young people (Wyn and White, 1997). Teenagers' agency is, however, persistently understated in schools and wider educational institutions (Mayall, 2002).

Recognizing active citizenship at school

One of the key themes in teenagers' experiences of citizenship within school is that of relevancy. Many participants valued subject matter that was of relevance to their current lives, as well as to their future status. This is essential to ensuring that teenagers' current status and place within society is not undermined. Furthermore, relevancy was also of importance to participants in relation to the transition from childhood to adulthood. Several valued such education particularly in relation to explaining age-specific legislation and key legal landmarks. Nevertheless, there was a certain degree of disaffection with the subject matter. Many participants believed that citizenship education had greater value for their future lives, thus echoing the notion of 'citizens-in-the-making'. Significantly, there was an important relationship between the way teenagers felt they were treated within such lessons and their engagement with the curriculum. The older participants felt they were viewed by teachers, the more engaged they were with citizenship. Respect for teenagers' status and a more egalitarian approach in the classroom has the potential to strengthen citizenship within schools and the wider community. Furthermore, such an approach may help to challenge a deeper, ingrained education culture which does not fully appreciate children and teenagers as citizens-in-the-present. More broadly, there were diverse understandings of the transferability of citizenship as a curriculum subject to the wider world. For those who could not envisage the relevancy of the subject to their communities, this may be a reflection of young teenagers' exclusion from mainstream politics, inciting attitudes such as 'what's the point in learning about voting when we can't do it?'. Others upheld the importance of being informed.

The second key factor influencing the 'effectiveness' of the citizenship curriculum relates to implementation and delivery. Many teenagers valued participatory methods of teaching. Within schools children and teenagers have little opportunity to shape their curricula. Alderson (2000b) suggests that children and young people become democratic citizens through practice. The school council provided a valuable space of citizenship for many teenagers, producing tangible and very real outcomes. It also allowed teenagers to voice their opinions, ensuring that teachers were able to make decisions based upon consultation rather than assumption. It was, at times, challenging to maintain an effective school council. Alderson suggests poor examples of citizenship in practice within schools have the potential to disengage teenagers. In this research, participants also provided examples of citizenship in practice through their own micro-geographies of citizenship within the playground. Through the distinct and explicit geographies of hanging out at school, exclusions and contestations of school spaces were highlighted. These challenges and conflicts occurred between teenagers as well as with members of staff. Analysis of the micro-politics of the informal school not only illustrates what teenagers learn from their own experiences, for example power relations and conflict, decision-making and negotiation, but also highlights the unequal power relationships between staff and students which do little to promote democracy in schools.

This analysis provides a strong case for developing a more fluid notion of citizenship in which children, teenagers and adults alike are represented as full citizens who, during their lives, engage in different forms of citizenship in different arenas. As Kingston argues with reference to post-16 citizenship education:

However little they [sic] might know of how their country ticks, many teenagers are doing quite a lot of what could be described as citizenship.

(2002: 50)

It is to the consideration of teenagers' own engagements with citizenship, outside the classroom, that the next chapter turns.

Chapter 5

Practising citizenship in the wider community

Introducing alternative understandings

In-depth interviews with participants regarding their engagement with citizenship commenced with a seemingly meaningless and unrelated question in order to establish rapport – 'Did you watch *Big Brother*[10] last night?' All participants replied positively and we engaged in dialogue over who would be the next to be evicted! Amidst discussions that the increase in television viewing has contributed to a decline in conventional civic engagement is the notion that (electoral) politics needs to adapt in order to counter voter apathy (see Putnam, 2000). Turner (2004) suggests that more people cast votes for the 2004 *Big Brother* eviction by telephone and text message than were placed in the 2001 general election at polling booths. Many of these *Big Brother* voters were teenagers. This example illustrates that, despite the notion of teenage apathy, many young people are engaged in alternative forms of (electoral) politics. Moreover, Roker *et al.*'s (1999) analysis of young people's voluntary and campaigning activities suggests that many young people *are* actively involved in, for example, single issue campaigns. These acts of engagement have a number of positive outcomes for young people's political development including the acquisition of skills, knowledge and confidence. This chapter is concerned with teenagers' own practices and experiences of citizenship. Looking beyond formal citizenship education within school and children-centred political institutions, such as youth forums, I explore the ways in which teenagers act as political agents and indeed citizens in their own spaces and communities.

Using several case studies the chapter highlights examples of young teenagers who have devised *creative spaces of citizenship* and resourceful ways in which to redefine and reconstruct everyday spaces and identities. To contextualize the spaces of citizenship that teenagers spend time in and value, I first explore geographies of hanging out within the community. This is followed by a more in-depth exploration of participants' interests and their subsequent effect on participation. Participants' creativity and citizenship in shaping their communities is then outlined through examples of teenagers' alternative modes of citizenship such as developing skate-park facilities, campaigning for the preservation of youth centres and carving out spaces in marginalized areas of their environments. Finally, young teenagers' own definitions of important facets of citizenship, namely 'community' and 'identity', are a focus. Many of these identifications challenge conventional understandings and are commonly associated with lifestyle-based communities of practice.

Recognizing active citizenship

Teenage geographies of hanging out within rural communities provide a context for teenagers' lived experiences outside school. As Lister *et al.* (2003) point out, belonging represents a 'thick' notion of citizenship which moves beyond simply being a member of a community, and Hall *et al.* (1999) argue that more contemporary, fluid understandings of citizenship focus on issues of belonging at the local level. Exploring teenagers' geographies of hanging out allows the examination of belonging, as well as participants' political actions within places significant to them. 'Hanging out', therefore, is also an important context for teenagers' relationship with citizenship. Subsequently, participants' interests and responsibilities are explored particularly in relation to their impact upon participation. Finally, the numerous ways in which many teenagers shape and claim everyday spaces within their communities will be highlighted as an important introduction to the notion of *creative spaces of citizenship*.

Claiming micro-spaces of citizenship

In the first questionnaire, participants described the places in which they regularly hang out. Table 2 outlines examples of the arenas noted in the questionnaire. Whilst they are loosely categorized into a typology, the blurred boundaries between such spaces must also be recognized. Indeed, these distinctions are not discrete, as 'claimed spaces' were often 'public spaces' and some 'public spaces' were occasionally more private than, for example, 'commercial spaces'.

There are, of course, limitations to requesting responses of this nature via a survey. Participants may, consciously or unconsciously, alter or hide the actual spaces they socialize in for a number of reasons. For example, they may wish not to disclose spaces that they value outside the adult gaze. Here, my position as an adult researcher and 'outsider' may have affected the extent to which respondents were willing to provide me with glimpses of their worlds. The survey did however reveal that public spaces were the arenas most commonly frequented by teenagers, closely followed by commercial spaces. Tranter and Pawson (2001) outline streetscapes as well as more wild settings as arenas in which children play and 'hang out'. Unlike

Table 2 Where do you socialize with friends?

Where do you hang out?	Number of times cited by participants	Examples
Private spaces	91	Own home Friend's home
Public spaces	177	Beach Park/green Woods Recreational ground Skate parks
Commercial spaces	166	Town Cinema Leisure centres Cafes Pubs/clubs
Claimed spaces	92	Streets Benches Other school's grounds Bus shelters Graveyards

the geographies of hanging out within school outlined in chapter 4, participants often had several regular locations within their local and wider communities. These different spaces were based upon a broader range of opportunities and activities than hanging out within the school (Matthews *et al.*, 2000b; Tucker and Matthews, 2001). Participants' or friends' homes were important places especially for those living in more isolated areas. Within the home, teenagers' bedrooms were significant spaces of both privacy and identity. Bob lives in a town where the majority of other teenage residents attend a different high school. He stays in his room most days after school, reading, watching television or videos. More isolated teenagers like Bob have less opportunity for social networks and so spend more time in their rooms:

> I don't go out after school because I have no friends in [town] but there's plenty to do in [town] when my friends come round.
> (Extract from Bob's diary)

Hanging out in the home is not just for those who are isolated from other teenagers. Funda describes her friend's house (see plate 3), isolated from adult gaze, as a secluded space for hanging out:

SUSIE: Where's that?
FUNDA: Um ... it's [boy's name] house ...
SUSIE: Oh right.

FUNDA: ... and cos he's got a massive, massive house we're all allowed up there so it's like a good place to be cos it's like it's a house far away from everything else and no one can hear if we get up to anything like ...

SUSIE: (Laughs)

FUNDA: ... music and what not.

(Group discussion, 2nd July 2002)

Secluded, private spaces are particularly important to Funda and her friends. She notes how the nocturnal activities of teenagers in her local town are under the surveillance of regular police patrols. To avoid such surveillance Funda often socializes in private spaces.

Many teenagers displayed what Faulks (2000) refers to as a post-modern or cosmopolitan approach to citizenship. This suggestion is not bound to closed political boundaries but is pluralistic in nature. Concurrently, local boundaries shape the everyday spaces of citizenship and belonging for teenagers, many of which are tied to the local. This does not, however, conflict with the notion of a post-modern citizenship, but rather upholds that in the immediate future citizenship will be acted out at the local level. Painter and Philo (1995) examine the exclusion from citizenship of those who seek 'safe havens' away from public space to express their identities comfortably. In these terms many teenagers 'claim spaces' away from adult surveillance in order to assert their autonomy and are often seen as a threat to adult-dominated public space (Matthews *et al.*, 2000a; 2000b), constructing 'underground geographies'. Claimed spaces were hugely important to teenagers' geographies of hanging out and citizenship. Claimed spaces are those which groups or individual teenagers have adopted as regular meeting places within their communities, and commonly include benches and bus stops (see also Hall *et al.*, 1999) (see plate 4). Such places are often simple features of the natural or built landscape, as Nikki highlighted:

SUSIE: How about are there any places that you've like claimed as your own?

NIKKI: Yeah we either go up near the pavilion or we sit down by the swings and that's like where we were but now all the like younger people have started coming over as well. It's just not the same.

SUSIE: Do you know why you chose those places?

NIKKI: Er ... I think it's just like cos it's quite close cos where I ... most of the people who go to [park] live in [town] anyway. It's somewhere in the middle of us lot.

SUSIE: Yeah.

NIKKI: So it's easier to go there.

(Group discussion, 2nd July 2002)

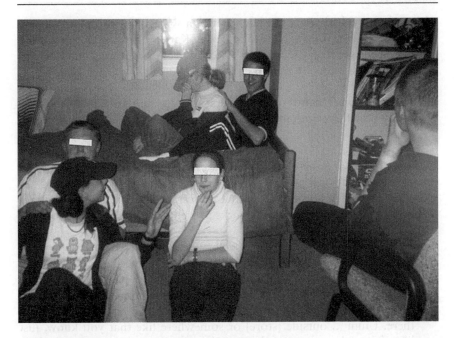

Plate 3 Hanging out at friends' houses, photographed by Funda

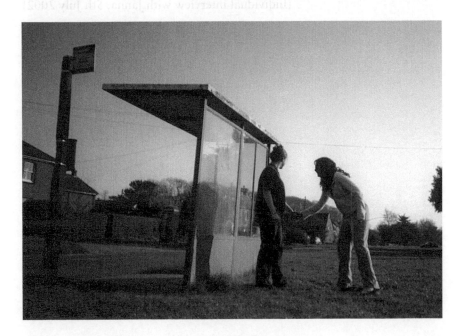

Plate 4 Hanging out at the bus stop, photographed by Matt

Although individual teenagers hang out in a wide variety of places, many had a particular favourite or regular space. Katie, for example, spends her time along the sea front (see plate 5). Meanwhile, Chloe carved out her own space in a bus station (see plate 6):

> I've taken one [photo] of the bus station because I seem to spend most of my time there with my mates.
>
> (Group discussion, 3rd July 2002)

Everyday spaces are, therefore, utilized for socializing and many such places are significant sites for groups of teenagers to gather prior to deciding the day's activities. These regular meeting places are also important in establishing and maintaining social networks as well as countering isolation:

> Where we know [town] quite well, we have different meeting places round [town] where like a whole twenty of us'll meet up and go wherever we're gonna go from there, so there is a couple of ... um ... the green is one of them. We all meet up there sometimes and ... there's a couple of car parks like the central car park in [town]. We meet up there. Umm ... outside [store] or somewhere like that you know, just like places where everyone knows where it is because you meet up there all the time.
>
> (Individual interview with Janna, 5th July 2002)

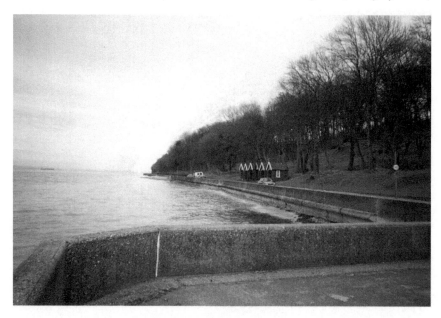

Plate 5 Hanging out along the sea front, photographed by Katie

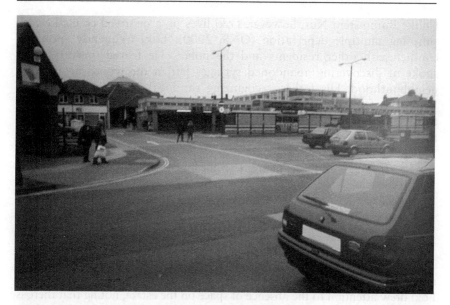

Plate 6 Hanging out in the bus station, photographed by Chloe

As chapter 6 will highlight, many teenagers are frustrated at the general lack of affordable and accessible facilities where they live and many do not have the means to travel. These everyday places, therefore, become highly significant to teenagers' lives. Furthermore, as Nikki suggests above, there is often competition for, and conflict over, particular sites by different groups of children and teenagers (Tucker and Matthews, 2001).

Some teenagers, for example, talked of carving out typically rural places. Rammstein Nut, a self-confessed tomboy, lives in a rural area with few neighbouring young people. Although she enjoys some spatial freedoms typically associated with 'growing-up' in a rural area, she also experiences much isolation. Despite this, Rammstein Nut makes her mark upon the rural landscape:

> I've made lots of treehouses and stuff (Laughs) ... and bases ... to pass my time ... Yeah. There's a caravan site ... it's like really boring but I've made some like bases and hideouts ... around. When my friends come round we can ... we go down there.
>
> (Individual interview, 2nd July 2002)

Although demonstrating a seemingly small impact upon her community, Rammstein Nut's example illustrates active decision-making over micro-spaces. This adoption of highly localized spaces is a relatively dominant theme within teenagers' discourses of hanging out (Tucker and Matthews, 2001). Loki also develops the notion of claiming specifically rural spaces.

Unlike Rammstein Nut, however, Loki lives on a deprived council estate suffering multiple deprivation (ONS, 2000). Loki frequently spoke of conflict with other residents and the police. He feared 'perverts' and spoke of discovering abandoned syringes left in the woods around his neighbourhood. His father, recognizing the local problems, often took Loki away from the estate in an attempt to prevent him from getting into trouble. Together they pursued relatively rural pursuits such as fishing and shooting:

> I go fishing with my Dad and I've got lots of little secret spots ... and I go shooting. Um ... around [estate] the only place is the field so I've got a little tree ... it's got a base in there ... hammock sort of thing and that's ours ... and that's it.
>
> (Group discussion, 3rd July 2002)

Through engagement in rural pursuits, Loki's father attempted to reconstruct a pure and idyllic childhood for his son, away from the estate. Furthermore, Loki drew attention to the absence of space on the estate, noting that there is only one area where he and his friends could create a space for themselves. The rural spaces that Loki visited with his father, therefore, became the arenas over which he had control, particularly as they were set aside from the police and neighbourhood surveillance on the streets of the estate.

In seemingly structured and organized activity spaces such as youth clubs, some teenagers also manage to carve out and claim their own spaces. Gumdrop goes to a youth club twice a week. Whilst there, she and her friends have created their own space within the building, seeking solace in a small area of corridor away from adult surveillance and the noise of the rest of the club (see plate 7).

> We just wanted somewhere where we could sit that was like ... cos it's quite hectic in youth club cos there's lots of people ... lots of stupid boys and um ... (Laughs) so we just want to go somewhere quiet where we can just sit and chat and the corridor's quite good for that.
>
> (Group discussion, 2nd July 2002)

After the club closes Gumdrop and her friends move location to their regular hangout outside the building (see plate 8).

Regularly socializing in the same spaces helps participants shape their communities. Kendal, for example, stated that he met his friends on a daily basis at his local skate park and, as will be revealed later in this chapter, had been actively involved in campaigning for the facility. Hanging out was not, however, always so static. Many participants spoke of a travelogue of socializing, starting in one place and moving round to others:

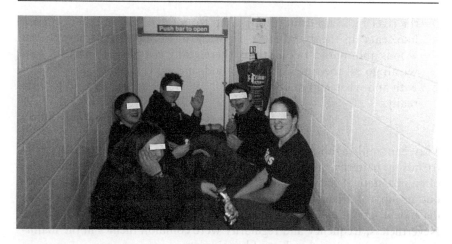

Plate 7 Claiming spaces, youth club, photographed by Gumdrop

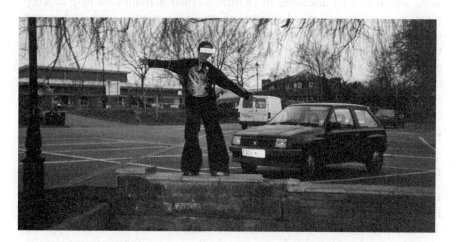

Plate 8 Hanging out outside the youth club, photographed by Gumdrop

KITTY SANDORAL: ... when I'm in [town] with my friends we tend to go to places like [name] rec and stuff. We just go sit on the swings and just like places like that. I mean we ... well we tend ... you can walk down a lane from up by [shop], we walk down there and we go and sit by the river down there.

SUSIE: Oh right.

KITTY SANDORAL: ... cos I mean it's by the road but you've got the river there and there's a pipe which we sit on which goes across the river so we sit there sometimes and um ... also down ... down, further down the river by ... up from [shop] ... up from the path there's a ... there's like seats up there and stuff. So we just go and sit up there in the woods and that ... I don't think there really is a place that's ... where we all go all the time. It's like Gumdrop said it depends on who I'm with and what we're doing and stuff like that but we just tend to drift really.

(Group discussion, 2nd July 2002)

Kitty Sandoral highlights how geographies of hanging out are shaped by friendship patterns. Several of the diary entries suggested that friendship is often in a state of flux. On different days participants spent time with various groups of friends. The spaces in which they socialized were often dependent upon which group of friends they were with at the time. Nevertheless, frequency and regularity were common themes in the majority of participants' geographies of hanging out.

Whilst teenagers' presence in public space does create the kinds of tensions which will be discussed in chapter 6, their activities do help to keep rural communities alive. Moreover, micro-level activities such as hanging out start to reveal the everyday encounters of the political. The places in which teenagers hang out are perhaps, to them, the most important spaces of citizenship. It is in these spaces that teenagers' political agency is demonstrated on a variety of scales. Such arenas are often dynamic and temporary, revealing the production and reproduction afforded to spatiality (Merrifield, 2000). The next section of this chapter details teenagers' involvement and participation in shaping their communities.

Citizen involvement

Bound to the notion of teenage apathy is the concern that young people are increasingly disengaged from political and community issues (Pretty, 1998). To some extent, findings in this research reinforce this idea with few participants involved in formal voluntary work. Putnam's (2000) influential work on social capital in American communities explores changes in civic engagement. One such measure of engagement, Putnam suggests, is the individualization of leisure time, with trends inferring an increase in home-based leisure pursuits such as watching television. Participants in this research demonstrated alternative forms of collective or communal engagement and citizenship through, for example, hanging out with friends, skateboarding (which can also be done individually), organized sports and youth clubs. Responses to the first survey revealed 'hanging out with friends' (76 per cent) and 'skateboarding/biking' (47 per cent) as the most popular pursuits and these were also amongst the least individualized activities (Weller, 2006a).

Several teenagers participated in team activities in a more conventional sense. Kitty Sandoral regularly plays in a local marching band:

> I do a lot of music stuff cos I play the clarinet and stuff. I need to get my grades up. I'm on about grade 5 or 6 at the moment so I like play in music centre wind band like at [school] on Saturday mornings and stuff like that.
>
> (Group discussion, 2nd July 2002)

Kitty Sandoral said that attending the band meetings was not only beneficial to her musical attainment but also gave her the opportunity to widen her social networks. Despite participating in this more traditional activity, she and her friends found ways of carving out their own spaces of citizenship during their time with the band. Kitty Sandoral highlighted two particular ways in which this was achieved. First, the band spends a considerable length of time travelling during the summer vacation, and so band members made additions to the minibus to make it more 'homely':

> ... inside [the] minibus cos we like it cos it's got comfy seats and stuff, and we started making it like a bit more homely with curtains ... and we've put loads of stuff cos we're in there so much ... like in the summer ...
>
> (Group discussion, 2nd July 2002)

Second, Kitty Sandoral and her friends challenged the rigidity of band rehearsals by establishing a secluded space away from adult gaze in which to hang out during practice:

> Yeah I mean we go and sit down there and stuff, but like at band ... they've got long grass at the back of the Jubilee hut where we go to play and we just go and sit in the long grass because you can't be seen and they call it WI [Women's Institute] meetings (Laughs) cos you just ... like sit and talk up there and stuff.
>
> (Group discussion, 2nd July 2002)

Many of the other teenagers involved in more in-depth elements of the research were members of sports teams, dance groups and theatre companies:

> Today after school I went to football training for my team [town] 2000.
>
> (Extract from Crateser's diary)

Although Crateser is actively involved in his local football team he does not equate this to community participation. In his diary he explicitly stated that he had no interest in his community. The categorization of participation utilized in this research was not synonymous with the views of some participants. Crateser's diary entries challenged my perceptions of what defines a space of citizenship. Indeed, Lister (1997b) highlights how individuals do not always recognize that their actions are political. Nevertheless, it is fundamental that teenagers' individual motivations are acknowledged in order to evaluate what constitutes citizenship. This is, of course, no more complex than the examination of adult perceptions of, and motivations towards, participation and citizenship. Moreover, Crateser's statements challenge whether it is legitimate to 'label' an activity an act of citizenship when it is perhaps not intended to be.

Funda provides a very different example, one where traumatic events can bring teenagers and the wider community together through an alternative mutual interest:

> ... we did get involved like when someone ... a girl in [town] got attacked. I think everyone got involved in that ... because like everyone ... everyone knows everyone and everyone knew the people that did it and everyone got involved in that and tried to help her out but that's about the only thing.
>
> (Group discussion, 2nd July 2002)

Funda's observation suggests that, whilst her town conforms to stereotypical ideas of rural life where 'everyone knows everyone else', these bonds are only temporary. Social cohesion only occurred, from Funda's point of view, as a response to the violent act committed on both the girl and, more broadly, the social space of the town.

When asked to name something that would make their community a better place, many participants cited tangible outcomes such as a new facility. Several teenagers, however, outlined wider issues, calling for greater social cohesion:

SUSIE: ... if you could suggest one thing to make your community better what would it be?

KENDAL: More events on our ... so it gets everybody closer together ...

SUSIE: Yeah.

KENDAL: ... everybody grows closer and becomes more family. That would be better cos there aren't too many ... there aren't that many events. Better to get everybody closer.

> (Group discussion, 4th July 2002)

Kendal highlighted the need for collective participation in order to build greater community bonds, which he hoped would be akin to bonds within a family. Many teenagers are, therefore, actively involved in their communities in a diverse range of ways and are by no means solely pursuing individualized, home-based activities.

Fundamentally, participants in the first survey called for a greater voice in local decision-making. Just under three-quarters (72 per cent; n = 425) wished to have the opportunity to voice their opinions on local issues, which suggests that a relatively sizeable proportion of respondents had no desire to be involved. In line with these figures a poll conducted by MORI (2001) also found that 71 per cent of 16–24 year-olds desired a greater say in decision-making. The questionnaire administered in this research did not enable participants to elaborate upon their answers, but in-depth discussions with several of these respondents did suggest a level of despondency. The belief that those in power would not act meaningfully upon the requests of young people deterred several teenagers from taking an interest in participation. The difference between boys' and girls' responses was not statistically significant. Furthermore, whilst these figures imply *intended* participation rather than *actual* participation, it is fundamental to consider the often unrecognized ways in which many teenagers already actively contribute to shaping their communities.

Citizen responsibilities

In much of this book I have argued for teenagers' rights to citizenship. As chapter 2 outlined, many understandings of citizenship also count 'duties' or 'responsibilities' as an important element. In the second questionnaire participants were asked to detail any responsibilities they felt they had in their communities. The most common response was respecting the environment (16 per cent; n = 172). This included keeping areas tidy, safe and free from vandalism:

> Don't vandalise things. Look after town.
>
> (Female, aged 14)

Several teenagers (9 per cent) suggested that their responsibility was to be a citizen and to help and to respect others:

> Look after people and the environment.
>
> (Female, aged 14)

> Being a helpful citizen.
>
> (Male, aged 15)

A few (7 per cent) believed it was their responsibility to behave well, abide by laws and not to be violent:

> Not getting into trouble.
>
> (Female, aged 15)

Other responsibilities outlined by a small minority included improving local life, having fun and taking part in sports events. Only 7 per cent explicitly stated that they did not have any responsibilities in their communities. Whilst this question was challenging to answer, many respondents were able to outline the contributions that they felt they should be making to their communities and so demonstrated their awareness of some form of 'active citizenship' at the local level. The next section explores examples of *creative spaces of active citizenship* within rural communities in order to move beyond participation in terms of hanging out to that which leaves a lasting impact upon the wider community.

Creative spaces of active citizenship

In 2000 two school boys took their local council to the High Court in order to save their football field from redevelopment (Price, 2000). As a result of their action they won the right to have their opinions taken into account. This illustrates one example of young people exerting their political agency over an issue important to them. In this study skateboarding and the development of skate parks was the most frequently cited form of participation. Other examples included the development of play areas, sports facilities, parks, youth clubs and more general improvements to existing facilities. On one level teenagers participate in short-term single events, although many of these experiences have had lasting impacts. On another level there is more long-term participation through the development and maintenance of skate parks. There are contestations and difficulties inherent in creating each of these spaces of citizenship.

Revitalizing rural communities

Over one-third (36 per cent; n = 133) of respondents in the second questionnaire had participated in their communities. The most popular form of involvement (22 per cent) was in a local campaign. Several teenagers (8 per cent) had been involved in planning a local event, for example, painting a mural; helping to maintain local rock concerts; or involvement in a bid for money to improve the local environment. Only a few respondents (7 per cent) were involved in voluntary work. Chapter 1 outlined Foster's (1997) critique of contemporary citizenship as a patriarchal construct. She suggests that the assignment of women to the private sphere renders their true access to formal (public) civic institutions problematic. In my research there was a significant statistical difference between girls' and boys' involvement, with boys more likely (44 per cent) to participate in their communities in activities such as skate-park campaigns, than girls (26 per cent) who were more likely to engage in voluntary work such as fundraising or helping out at a local youth club (Weller, 2006a).

Two participants, Matt and Kat, live in an isolated village, which comprises one relatively affluent part and one more deprived estate ranked amongst the top 30 per cent of wards in terms of multiple deprivation in England (ONS, 2000). The area has few facilities for teenagers and limited connections to other towns and villages. Matt highlighted an important space where teenagers regularly hang out (see plate 9):

> Went down the busie in [village] and played out with my friends. Later on went back down busie.
>
> (Extract from Matt's diary)

Matt referred to the 'busie', a disused bus stop, every day in his week-long diary as an important space for gathering and socializing (Weller, 2006a). Kat reinforces the significance of the space:

> The 'busie' is a good place. We all hang out ... and say how we feel about people. It is the only thing we can really do because there is nothing to do in [village]. We have some fields but no park or anything like that.
>
> (Extract from Kat's diary)

The 'busie' was also a symbolic site of citizenship for Kat as she had taken on an important role in both saving 'the busie' from demolition by the local

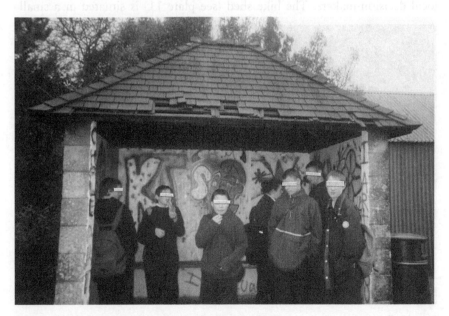

Plate 9 Hanging out in the 'busie', photographed by Kat

authority, and using a council grant to reshape the space (see plate 10) (Weller, 2006a):

> The bus shelter was going to get knocked down because everyone was writing horrible words in it and none of the people round the estate really liked it so we made the decision that we were going to keep it tidy and we were going to paint it so all the graffiti [was covered up] and so the council gave us money to buy the spray paint.
>
> (Group discussion, 4th July 2002)

The 'busie' demonstrates not only teenagers' engagement with citizenship at the local level but illustrates ways in which very real and positive attitudes by local decision-makers can promote teenagers' participation in their communities. This is particularly valuable in an area where there has been notable conflict between the activities of some teenagers and other local residents. In Kat's village, involving children and teenagers in local decision-making has now been taken a step further with the establishment of a forum where regular dialogue may well lead to further improvements in the village's facilities (Weller, 2003; 2006a). Positive examples of support for young people's self-directed projects do exist in other countries. Kjørholt (2004), for example, details a national grants scheme for children living in Norway.

On the other side of the Island, Kimbo and Kaz discussed a similar space to the 'busie', one which is of great significance to many local teenagers and one in which they have actively participated in saving, in collaboration with local decision-makers. The bike shed (see plate 11) is situated in a small

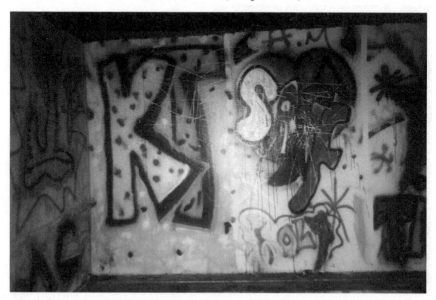

Plate 10 Creative spaces, the 'busie', photographed by Kat

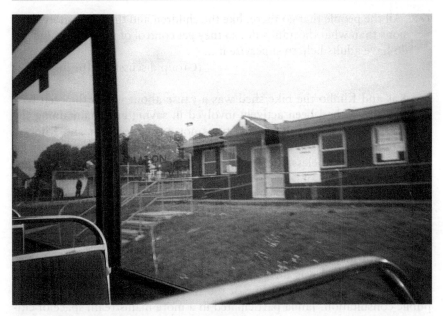

Plate 11 The bike shed, photographed by Kaz

town, featuring in the top 25 per cent of wards suffering multiple deprivation in England (ONS, 2000). The space was not only a social arena but, again, a place in which they had participated as active citizens, saving the facility from permanent closure and raising funds:

KIMBO: The bike shed is like ... on Wednesdays there's like food there and people go down there to play pool and stuff.
KAZ: It's like a youth club.
SUSIE: Oh right, yeah.
KAZ: Everyone just goes in there and chills.
KIMBO: Yeah I've been involved with the bike shed. We had to do this thing cos it was going to get shut down ...
SUSIE: Yeah.
KIMBO: ... so it got shut down for a little while but it's open now. We like decided everything. They used to build bikes there and that but they don't no more.
KAZ: Yeah I used to always like get on TV ...
SUSIE: Really.
KAZ: Yeah, Children in Need ...
SUSIE: Oh excellent! So when you were making decisions over the bike shed did you have quite a lot of control over it or ... did you have what you and your friends wanted?

KAZ: All the people that go there, like the children and that have more decisions than what the adults do, so they get control of it basically. But we
do have adults help to supervise it ...

(Group discussion, 4th July 2002)

For Kat and Kimbo the bike shed was a cause about which they felt pas-
sionate, and so had been actively involved in saving and maintaining the
space for future use. Such contributions not only affect Kat and Kimbo's
lives and experiences of citizenship but also have an impact for the wider
community. Nevertheless, the 'busie' and the bike shed are, however, specifically teenage spaces of citizenship.

Janna told of her involvement in a bid for a regeneration grant for her
seaside town. Again, Janna lives in an area suffering from multiple deprivation, within the top 20 per cent of deprived wards in England (ONS, 2000).
She was specifically asked to represent local children and young people in
her town in meetings regarding the bidding process. She explained that,
whilst the proposal was unsuccessful, local decision-makers were keen to
find other funds to resolve some of the issues and ideas raised during the
public consultation. Janna participated in a more mainstream space of citizenship within the realms of adult decision-making. In this space she
generally felt listened to, although she acknowledged that not all of her
ideas were considered:

SUSIE: Do you think your ... your opinions were listened to?
JANNA: Er yeah they were. Cos ... um ... I actually I told them so, and people asked questions about them so I reckon people did listen but not
much was done about it, even though they did listen.
SUSIE: Did you have a discussion or did you fill in a questionnaire or something ...?
JANNA: Er ... no actually it was a ... I was invited to a big meeting ...
SUSIE: Oh right ...
JANNA: ... like with lots of important people and stuff. The mayor and
stuff. It was ... it was quite nerve racking but I'm like used to speaking
out loud cos I'm into drama and um ... it was ... I reckon they did listen they just didn't take, perhaps everything into consideration that I
had said.

(Individual interview, 5th July 2002)

In addition to Janna's involvement in a public consultation, as we have seen
in chapter 4, she is also her class representative on the school council.
Janna, therefore, has much experience of engaging in more formal spaces of
citizenship. Nevertheless, she also exerts her political agency in more radical
forms of civic engagement:

JANNA: Oh there was this huge ... there's been ... recently there was this huge thing about umm ... a local ... I don't know what you would call it ... umm ... a [theatre] do ... like a gig every month ...

SUSIE: Yeah.

JANNA: Umm ... 'Battle of the Bands' they did and stuff like that, and then about a couple of weeks ago there was like 'oh no we're gonna shut it down'.

SUSIE: Really?

JANNA: There was a huge protest saying, you know, that there is actually nothing to do, and they complain that people my age go out and get drunk ...

SUSIE: Yeah.

JANNA: ... but what do they expect us to do when there's nothing else to do.

SUSIE: Yeah.

JANNA: Do you see what I mean?

SUSIE: Yeah.

JANNA: So when they were closing that down there was a huge protest and a lot of people turned up to ... I think to say that they didn't think that it was a good idea to close it down. Luckily they haven't!

(Individual interview, 5th July 2002)

Formal and informal spaces of citizenship are not mutually exclusive and the boundaries between such spaces are often dynamic. Kat, Matt, Kaz, Kimbo and Janna all cite examples of the ways in which teenagers individually and collectively shape and revitalize their environments despite not being seen as full citizens in terms of more conventional understandings of citizenship. Much of this participation has some degree of collaboration with local decision-makers. Bob Stevens and his friends, however, have built temporary bike ramps at the bottom of his street (see plate 12). He argued that, whilst there has been conflict over the space with other local residents, the users demonstrate responsible behaviour. In return they expect respect from other residents, although this is not always given:

BOB STEVENS: ... we have to make our own ramps.

SUSIE: Is that your road where you live?

BOB STEVENS: Yeah. My house is just there.

SUSIE: How do like other people in the road feel about you making ramps at the end? Are they quite happy?

BOB STEVENS: There's this person here that always complains. He phones the police up. [My friend] ... he jumped into this ... umm ... and there was like a bottle, and it broke on his foot.

(Group discussion, 3rd July 2002)

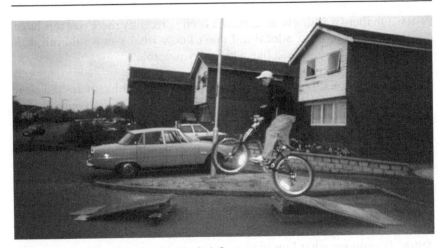

Plate 12 Bike ramps, photographed by Bob Stevens

Bob Stevens' example details an attempt to revitalize his community by providing a facility for local teenagers. The bike ramp that he created was neither praised nor respected by some of the other local residents. The development of skate parks and skateboarding are also significant as *creative spaces of citizenship*.

Skate parks

The importance of skateboarding to many participants in my research emerged during the pilot of the first questionnaire. One explanation for the strong skateboarding culture on the Island is its relationship to the more established surf culture. Such a link is referred to by Borden (2001), who notes that skateboarding in the 1960s and 1970s was principally undertaken by surfers. Significant both as a sport and a group identity, the presence of skateboarding within communities on the Island created both spaces of citizenship and arenas of conflict. Acts of involvement such as campaigning for skate-park facilities often go unrecognized in statistical analysis and, therefore, exacerbate the notion of teenage apathy particularly for boys (Roker *et al.*, 1999; Weller, 2006a). Giddens (2000b) notes changes in voluntarism from traditional recognitions to those based on self-help. One example which reflects this shift is the popular involvement in developing skate-park facilities. Primarily carried out by boys, skate parks are one way in which many participants exercised their political agency within a contemporary space. Skate parks are designated sites where ramps have been constructed in order to carry out stunts. Over the past few years there has been an increase in the number of sites constructed particularly by local authorities, some of which view skate parks as a remedy to the much disputed 'youth problem'.

Kendal has actively campaigned for a skate park in his town (see plate 13), raising both finances and awareness. Since it has been built, Kendal has been helping to maintain the skate park's website:

KENDAL: We all helped the skaters and stuff. We helped to raise money and stuff.

SUSIE: How did you do that? How did you go about that?

KENDAL: We just like ... we got jars and stuff and put them in shops ... like in the skate shop in [town] put a jar in there for people and we just ... people signed petitions to like ... we went round shops signing petitions so we could get it done. Hopefully we're getting another bit done on the skate park ...

SUSIE: Really?

KENDAL: Yeah so that's quite cool. At the moment me and my dad are like doing a website for it ... we've just recently had a competition down there and so there's some pictures on that.

SUSIE: ... Who started it all off?

KENDAL: What the ...

SUSIE: The skate park.

KENDAL: Someone called [girl's name].

SUSIE: Is that like somebody independent? It wasn't the council or anything like that?

KENDAL: No ... she just ... well it was just her and a bunch of skaters that just wanted to build a park so she just ... I think she got a lottery grant ...

(Group discussion, 4th July 2002)

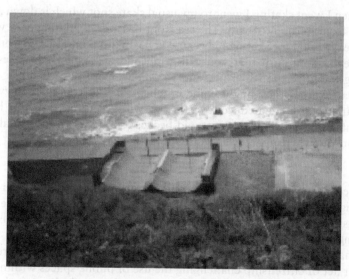

Plate 13 Creative spaces, the skate park, photographed by Kendal

Kendal's commitment to his local skate park is long term and he demonstrates both his rights and responsibilities as a citizen by continuing to campaign for the maintenance of the park (Weller, 2006a). Kendal has not only actively contributed to shaping his local environment but has also encouraged others to be involved. Matt, a friend of Kendal's, is keen to see a skate park in his village and is also prepared to participate in its development. This is significant for, as Roker *et al.* (1999) highlight, friends and peers are important in (dis)encouraging participation. Matt, however, presents a challenge to the bounded nature of citizenship within a skate park. Similar to children working on an environmental quality consultation project in California, who demonstrated their autonomous capacity as political actors by reconstructing knowledge they had gathered during the consultation to tear down a fence surrounding their apartments (Salvadori, 2001), many skateboarders like to skate on the street. This is often against the wishes of other local residents. Affording teenagers the opportunity to pursue their interest only within bounded spaces can lead to further conflict. When skating on the street, Loki is often challenged by some local residents and questioned as to why he is not skating in a designated skate park. Loki imitated a 'typical' objector:

> Yeah, it's like 'Well go over the skate park. You've got a perfectly good skate park there. Why do you skate here?'
>
> (Group discussion, 3rd July 2002)

Kendal echoed Loki's views:

> When I went skating I went to my usual skate spot which is down at the sea front in [home town]. The sea front has a dry paddling pool which is really good for skating in because you can jump into it. The front has a really long curb that you can grind and a couple of benches and ledges. I love the sea front, and I don't want to have it taken away because a new law might come in which says 'if you skate anywhere apart from designated skate spots you will get a fine and your board confiscated!' I think this is stupid because soon we will not be able to skate anywhere apart from skate spots.
>
> (Extract from Kendal's diary)

Some teenagers struggled against regulation in public space by exercising their 'right to dissent' through street skating. Matt's photograph (see plate 14) illustrates the reconstruction of space in his village through skateboarding using street signs, bus stops and walls (Weller, 2003).

In many ways, this alternative reconstruction of public space presents another act of citizenship challenging the use of public spaces within rural communities. In between the development of formal skate parks and

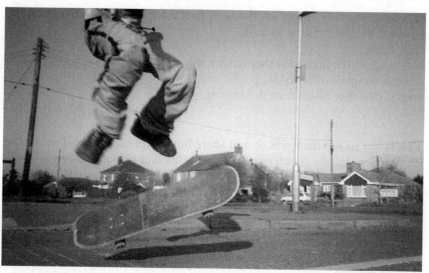

Plate 14 Reconstruction of village space, photographed by Matt

informal street skating lies the creation of informal skate-park areas where skaters have built home-made ramps. Kendal illustrated the dynamic nature of local spaces:

> I hung out at [village] skate park. It is a playground which has been converted into a park by the local skaters. There are loads of home-made ramps 'n' rails which are really cool and skatable.
>
> (Extract from Kendal's diary)

Kendal's example shows the temporal nature and interchangeability of spaces, and highlights Lefebvre's (1991) notions surrounding flows and collisions between different spaces, which when combined produce 'present space' (Merrifield, 2000). As a legitimate space of citizenship, skate parks have not only become an option for mitigating the problems of isolation and lack of facilities, but local decision-makers' resolution to build them has demonstrated a highly essentialist understanding of teenagers' needs. These 'top-down' developments were often built with little consultation and failed to tap into the knowledge, expertise, values and networks that made teenagers' own self-directed projects successful (Weller, 2006a; see also Woolley, 2006). Participation in skate parks and skateboarding more generally is, however, dominated by boys. Many girls discussed the lack of facilities relating to their interests (see also Morrow, 2003) and their exclusion from such masculinized spaces. Kat, Kaz and Kimbo noted the neglect of both girls and young children:

KAT: Like cos most things, say the skate park, that's really for boys so there's nothing like for girls to do ...

KAZ: Yeah.

KAT: And all the little kids they can't really go in the skating ramps cos it's too dangerous for them.

KIMBO: Cos they might hurt themselves.

(Group discussion, 4th July 2002)

This is not to say that girls do not skate but serves merely to illustrate the stereotypes placed upon teenagers. The rights and responsibilities inherent within citizenship are multilayered within the context of skate parks. As skaters, Kendal and Matt have demonstrated the ways in which many participants assume responsibility for their skate parks, although they are afforded few rights outside that arena (Weller, 2006a). Locally, skate parks have attracted much attention because several have been built and later vandalized. The following web-board discussion highlighted conflict within the community:

> First contributor: All very well having a skateboard park but are you going to look after it? We got one for the kids at [town]. Do the kids look after it? No they don't. Smash bottles. Fence has been ripped apart. And still the kids came down the bay with there [sic] skateboards damaging the seats and kerbstones.
>
> (iwight web forum, Adult, 2nd July 2003)

> Second contributor: In general skate parks are looked after very well indeed by skate boarders/bladers etc. who actually use the parks. The problems that arise around these areas are 90 per cent or more associated [mainly caused] by people that do not skate nor do they congregate in these areas when these parks are being used as is intended. Being an island there are limitations to facilities that are available for everyone that lives here, there is always the chance that someone will not use facilities as they are intended. Please do not blame without proof.
>
> (iwight web forum, 2nd July 2003)

The first contributor blames skateboarders for not respecting the facility, perhaps reinforcing the notion that all teenagers skate and are irresponsible. The second contributor retorts by suggesting that skateboarders do take responsibility for such parks and that conflict lies with those who do not use the park for its intended purpose. Skate parks and related skateboarding serve as an important example of the way in which teenagers actively contribute to shaping their communities, whether this is seen positively or negatively. When skate parks are built for the purposes of solving the 'youth problem' and regulating teenagers' use of space, their status as an arena for citizenship is brought into question. Nevertheless, spaces such as skate parks reveal the often hidden geographies of citizenship, not just in terms of practical participation but on a much deeper level of identity and belonging. These complexities of social identity are not only mapped out on many spatial scales, but are influenced profoundly by locality, peers and family networks (Weller, 2003).

Recognizing alternative citizen identities and communities

As this chapter has revealed, participants often demonstrated more fluid, post-modern practices of citizenship which reinforce Faulk's (2000) notion that in the immediate future (post-modern) citizenship will be acted out at the local level. Dominant understandings of citizenship, outlined in chapter 2, focus on the relationship between the individual and the nation-state which implicitly excludes young teenagers in a number of important contexts, for example, through the realm of paid work and through more mainstream mechanisms for political participation. For many participants citizenship was much more relevant at both the local and global levels.

Participants' identification with 'community' was complex and for many teenagers spaces of citizenship were often more significant at the micro-level, although reference was made to more global elements of citizenship. Indeed, several participants challenged the classification of the research site as 'rural'. Rather than conceiving of rurality through the lens of public narrative, many defined their communities through ontological narrative. Participants' challenges to institutional definitions of rurality demonstrate one of the ways in which teenagers construct their communities and surroundings as spaces of citizenship. Building upon discussions of teenagers' micro-spaces of citizenship two key examples are outlined in the following section which illustrate the ways in which participants challenged notions of 'belonging' and 'identity' as they are often portrayed in dominant understandings of citizenship. First, the myriad and often contested group identities which illustrate teenagers' sense(s) of belonging in unconventional spaces of citizenship are explored. Second, teenagers' engagement within cyberspace is highlighted as one potential means of practising citizenship in a more global arena.

Carving out diverse group identities

Integral to the consideration of teenagers' citizenship is the relationship between citizenship and identity. There is growing recognition that identity is a central element of citizenship (Cogan, 2000; Lister *et al.*, 2003), although many Western governments fear that this relationship is becoming less concerned with the nation-state (Lawson, 2001). Teenagers revealed the dynamics of spaces of citizenship through complex and often contested identities. Since the French Revolution, citizenship has been bound to cultural discourses of the nation-state. Such a union, Faulks (2000) argues, is not so relevant within post-modernity. In contradiction to Helve and Wallace's (2001) summation that children's identities are principally state-based, the opinions and experiences of participants were rarely expressed in terms of the nation-state (or European Union), except with respect to disillusion with, for example, the government (Weller, 2003). Instead, participants related to the local. Morrow (2000) suggests the creation of alternative communities by teenagers is, in some cases, a reaction to the exclusion that they feel from the wider world.

Belonging was often identified in terms of difference between teenagers, which reinforces Brown's (1997) notions of dynamic social identities in a radical citizenship (Weller, 2003). Putnam (2000) also highlights the increase in small group membership in the USA, terming the increase as the 'quiet revolution'. Bob, a skater, describes the signatures of local youth subcultures by explaining his interpretations of the social groups, the tensions and divisions:

BOB: Townies just sit on the bins outside McDonalds, and wear Adidas and Nike and stuff like that all the time.
SUSIE: Is there quite a lot of rivalry between the skaters and the townies?
BOB: Yeah.
SUSIE: Are there any other groups there?
BOB: There's the BMXers and the goths.
SUSIE: So there's lots of rivalry between all those groups?
BOB: No. Umm ... the skaters get on with the goths and the BMXers, so it's just there's townie-goths that like walk round pretending ... going 'Oh yer I'm a goth' but they're wearing Adidas and all that ... and there's townies that wear Adidas on skateboards, which gets on my nerves and there's townie-BMXers as well. Townies just act like they're like us and that's why they get on my nerves.

(Individual interview, 4th July, 2002)

Bob's example contests both adult constructions of social networks and political identities as well as demonstrating the complexity of teenagers' identities. Importantly, Bob highlights how such groups are not always distinct and indeed boundaries between and within groups are blurred. 'Townies' step across into the world of skateboarders and BMXers, and by doing so demonstrate the dynamic move in and between identities, often complying to acceptable lifestyle choices (Wyn and White, 1997; Weller, 2003; 2006a). Such groups are not unique to the research site and indeed,

Haydon (2002) takes a national look referring to such groups as 'tribes'. It is, therefore, particularly fruitful to draw upon Maffesoli's notion of *tribus,* or post-modern tribes whose sense of identity, 'state of mind' (1996: 98) and lifestyle are more fluid than conventional understandings of (youth) subcultures (see also Bennett, 1999; Weller, 2006a). Concurrently, group rivalry can render such identities discrete. Kitty Sandoral discusses some of the tensions between different groups of teenagers relating much of the conflict to difference:

> And they don't all get on with each other and there's a lot of like ... that's what it's like everywhere. Cos it's just different people are into different things and they just think ... there's a lot of people rivalry and a lot of people think different things and stuff like that. So it would be better if we were all more together.
>
> (Group discussion, 2nd July 2002)

Belonging to a group is a process of inclusion and exclusion. Some teenagers become members of one group as a safety measure against other groups (Haydon, 2002). Such groups are not synonymous with gangs. Being part of a group entails adopting an identity but does not necessarily involve hanging out with everyone else who has a similar identity. For example, not all skaters hang out together.

Place is highly significant to the development of identities (Vanderbeck and Dunkley, 2003). Kitty Sandoral suggests that all such groups have specific geographies within the community and spaces in which they exert their own forms of citizenship. These are marked by signatures such as clothing, music and the activities that different groups pursue:

KITTY SANDORAL: They're [townies] more into like ... it's different types of like shops and where they hang out and who they hang out with and they're more affected by what they look like and who they hang out with more than what they want to do and stuff. They're the sort of people which you do tend to see down [town] esplanade wearing very short skirts and high heels and basically just acting like prostitutes and smoking and drinking and stuff, they're sort of townies. And the foot-baller boys who just tend to think of like 'oh I have to look like a certain footballer' to fit in sort of thing. That's what I mean by town-ies.

SUSIE: So what kind of places do townies hang out in then?

KITTY SANDORAL: I figured it out ... um ... all the surfers and skaters go to [town] to get stoned at the weekend, and all the um ... townies go to [town] to get drunk and stuff ... Yeah cos they've got all the night clubs and stuff and they like listen to different types of music.

(Group discussion, 2nd July 2002)

Many participants described townies in terms of their identification with global brand names. For teenage participants in this research 'townies' were the most ostracized group as many felt they build their identity upon fashion brands and consumerism (Weller, 2006a). This identification is in itself a derivative of citizenship commonly associated with radical citizenship (Isin and Wood, 1999).

Kitty Sandoral also constructs most of the groupings she discusses as 'other' and does not place herself within any group other than her local marching band. Whilst many boys identified themselves with groups of skateboarders or BMXers, girls were less likely to discuss belonging along these lines other than hanging out occasionally with members of certain groups. Instead, many girls discussed friendship bonds and breakdowns principally with other girls both inside and outside of school. This echoes Morrow's (2000) study in which girls tended to refer to close or best friends, whereas boys were more likely to list several or many friends. Conflict over difference was, however, more apparent between groups of teenagers and other local residents. Many groups explicitly consist of young people. The greatest conflict has arisen between skateboarders and other members of the community, and as a result the legitimacy of skateboarders' activities has been questioned and they have become synonymous with deviant youth:

> I'm constantly hearing out where I live in [town], people are moaning and groaning endlessly about the kids hanging around down there by the sports centre ... umm ... you know, they're on skateboards cos there's a great little sort of, terracey car park there, so you can, you can escape from level to level and have a great time. But clearly, for some reason, even people that don't live there, that drive past, it irritates the hell out of them.
>
> (Presenter, Isle of Wight radio phone-in, 6th June 2003)

This attribution of deviancy, one contributor on a local web discussion suggests, is unjust:

> It is commonly presumed that skaters are the scum and the reason for most youth crime. It is not considered that skaters are actually pursuing a sport/hobby and are trying to improve their own skills at something. Instead when 'people' decide to throw the blame, they should consider the persecution skaters get from the non-skateboarding community of the same age. Perhaps it should be considered what these adolescents do to entertain themselves in their spare time?
>
> (iwight web forum)

These diverse groups and spaces of citizenship represent the somewhat disputed notion of 'radical citizenship', common in late modernity with the fragmentation and eclecticism of society. Isin and Wood's (1999) discussion of the proliferation of group identities highlights that not only do experiences within groups vary greatly along social fractures such as gender and sexuality, but that in many cases such groups are actively seeking connectedness and solidarity. Whilst participants in my research provide examples of fragmentation along new citizenship identities, many teenagers are forming groups which unite particularly along the lines of common interests. Indeed, Smith et al. (2002) discovered a similar, hidden geography of shared interest groups in rural New Zealand. Such localized citizen identities, therefore, have some degree of replication globally. Moreover, as Isin and Wood note:

> While academic and non-academic populism emphasises fragmented identities, the new social movements can be seen as efforts to redefine and reconstitute identity through political and discursive struggles over group rights and values.
>
> (1999: 154)

Arguably post-modern discourses provide a more appropriate lens through which to examine the fragmented and ruptured identities described by many teenagers than do writings concerning subculture(s) prevalent in the 1970s and 1980s (Watt, 1998). Indeed it is also fruitful to draw upon Wenger's (1998) notion of 'communities of practice'. Identity, Wenger believes, comes about through practice, with individuals defining themselves through participation, familiarity, past experiences and future plans. Communities of practice are those in which individuals are able to demonstrate competency, have full membership and understand and engage with one another (see also Weller, 2006a). The group dynamics outlined by participants sheds new light on definitions of belonging, community and identity, reinforcing the need for more fluid understandings of citizenship.

Potential arenas for global citizenship

The use of the internet by children and teenagers has stimulated a plethora of debate for many academics (see Bingham et al., 1999; Valentine and Holloway, 2001; Holloway and Valentine, 2003). Cyberspace presents an interesting challenge to concepts of 'citizenship' and 'community' in that interactions and exchanges take place in non-physical space. For many teenagers in this research cyberspace provides a seemingly viable means of overcoming the physical isolation of living in a rural area, as well as participating in a number of arenas of debate and local democracy. In open discussion several teenagers, principally girls, drew attention to the significance of internet chat rooms, messenger services and text messaging in their lives (Weller, 2006a). Messenger services allow participants to chat only to chosen friends. Chloe and Katie illustrate the significance of messenger services in maintaining friendships across the Island, as well as providing them with something to do:

KATIE: There's not much to do in [town] ...
CHLOE: No.
KATIE: ... so I just like go on the internet most nights ...
SUSIE: ... do you use chat rooms to communicate with people that way?
CHLOE: I don't use chat rooms as such but we have like a messenger service ...
SUSIE: Oh yeah, yeah ...
CHLOE: ... we use them to talk to our friends.
SUSIE: So you chat with friends.
CHLOE: Yeah.
SUSIE: Is that cos ... um ... do you chat with friends on the Island?
CHLOE: Yeah.
SUSIE: Is it cos they live in different places or ...?
CHLOE: Yeah.
KATIE: Yeah.
CHLOE: I speak to my friends from [town] ...
KATIE: Yeah. It's easier.
SUSIE: Is that cos you're quite spread out?
KATIE: Yeah.
CHLOE: Yeah. Not all ... you can't like everyday or every weekend phone them or go and see them so it's um ... a really good way of communicating cos most people nowadays have it.

(Group discussion, 3rd July 2002)

The school in which this research was undertaken has an intake of students from across the Island (Weller, 2006a). Friendships and social networks created during school were sometimes not easily transferable to the wider community, in terms of face-to-face interaction. Some teenagers spend up to two hours travelling home after school, primarily due to unintegrated transport. The internet and text messaging allow the distance between location and social interaction to be compressed (Laegran, 2002). Valentine and Holloway (2001) put forward the notion of 'extensibility', where distance is overcome through technology:

KITTY SANDORAL: But a lot of ... texting and stuff it's good cos you can keep in contact with them. I was having a conversation with my friend who lives down in Devon and I only see her like twice a year ...
SUSIE: Yeah.
KITTY SANDORAL: ... and we write to each other and stuff like that but we can keep contact like ... if she's watching an interesting programme we

can like 'oh turn the TV on' and stop and have a conversation about television.

GUMDROP: Yeah that's the thing about texting it's like instant so it's like if you're on holiday or something or doing something you can text away and say 'I'm blah, blah, blah, I'm blah, blah, blah'. Do you know what I mean?

(Group discussion, 2nd July 2002)

Cyberspace, therefore, has the potential to open up new spaces of citizenship for teenagers that are not bound to the nation-state. The information age has also reshaped citizens' relationship with rights and responsibilities (Giddens, 2000b), creating a global citizenship. Freie (1998) argues that community in cyberspace is implicitly counterfeit and refers to users as 'netizens'. Such networks, used to overcome geographical and emotional problems of isolation, are criticized by Freie for being undemocratic, exclusive and creating distanced relationships. Communities in cyberspace are principally commercial enterprises unlike democratic systems within what Freie terms genuine community, which is inclusive in that everyone has a stake in society. The extent, however, to which this stake is equal is highly contentious. Cyberspace, Freie continues, is also inherently exclusive. Whilst prejudices based upon class, gender or race may not be so prevalent, exclusion is founded upon access. The internet is centred only upon the communication aspect of community. Emotions and gestures are hard to convey, Freie suggests, in a way which harbours genuine community. Nevertheless, for some, the internet has opened up new avenues of participation and citizenship. Whilst numerous web forums exist relating to Island issues, including those for teenagers, Richard uses a forum on the local government website to voice his opinions and to interact with adults:

I think this web-board is a good way to communicate to the adult population, to be listened to. Most teenagers are judged on their appearance and this is why a lot of them are ignored or they are considered incompetent of understanding etc.

(iwight web forum, Richard, aged 17, posted 12th February 2003)

Rather than the creation of pseudo-citizens, where identities are fluid and sometimes false, Richard believes the use of the internet through media tools such as web forums allows teenagers to contribute to local debate without being judged by their appearance. Indeed, age is often not disclosed. Whilst Richard's experiences are not widespread, the use of cyberspace in enabling participation at the local, national and global levels is compelling, and rather disputes Odone's (2002) claim that children and young people are losing the ability to interact socially as a result of their fascination with cyberspace.

Moreover, many participants also considered the global dimensions of citizenship and potential connections with other young people across the world, as Janna highlights:

> ... you know there's young people half way across the world, like in America who are probably saying exactly the same thing as I am whereas they have got the money and everything ... and they've got the things that I want around them but they want more. It would be quite interesting to see what they have and what we have in comparison.
>
> (Individual interview, 5th July 2002)

These two key areas of citizenship and identity, coupled with examples of teenagers' practice at the local level, highlight what Isin and Wood (1999) refer to as the 'radical democratic citizen' composed of multiple layers of belonging and identity. For young teenagers this is still problematic because, whilst I have demonstrated the eclectic ways in which teenagers exert their citizenship and political agency as individuals and within groups, this is still outside mainstream democratic systems. These actions, therefore, are largely unrecognized by local decision-makers as active contributions to community life.

Active 'radical' citizens

The engagements with citizenship outlined in this chapter were commonly at the micro-level. Whilst some authors such as Flew (2000) have been rather dismissive of small-scale acts of citizenship, it is at the micro-level that many teenagers become interested and engaged in political issues and projects. Participants detailed, through the everyday places in which they hung out, their political actions as shapers and creators of local spaces of citizenship. This is not to say that the kinds of places that participants claimed and shaped were not under the watchful eye of the local panopticon, but that these sites were important places for meeting and establishing links with friends. This, in a sense, defies the notion that individualization is fostering an increase in solitary pursuits (for example, Putnam, 2000). Rather, the spaces in which participants spent their 'free time' were complex and dynamic, and ranged from collective socialization to spending time alone at home.

Through the shaping of micro-geographies, many participants challenged the notion of teenage apathy, and instead established themselves as committed political actors through developing and redeveloping areas within their communities. Much of this political action centred upon creating spaces for their own age group, whom they felt were afforded few facilities. Through campaigning for skate parks, revitalizing new spaces to hang out and maintaining old facilities, several participants demonstrated a somewhat radical approach to citizenship. Several also indicated the construction of citizenship identities along new lines of distinction, thus challenging ideas assigned to them. These groupings, centred upon lifestyle choice, were themselves fractured and dynamic. Many teenagers not only constructed their own forms of 'othering' between and within such groups but also questioned their status and legitimacy. It is likely that if this study was replicated in more cosmopolitan urban areas different citizen identities and affiliations would have been described which would reinforce the need for more fluid understandings of the key components of citizenship.

The spaces which participants occupied were not uncontested. The example of the popular phenomenon of skateboarding presents an interesting paradox. Whilst campaigning for and developing skate-park facilities was a prime example of active citizenship, the subsequent development of other skate parks in the area was seldom informed by consultation with teenagers. Indeed, many participants, particularly girls, saw the emergence of local-authority-developed skate parks as both a misguided solution to the 'youth problem' and, moreover, essentializing teenagers' needs and interests. For some skaters, the bounded nature of a skate park contested the legitimacy of access to other more public spaces and questioned the skate park as a meaningful space of citizenship.

The sum of these individual and collective political actions, if they are understood as acts of citizenship, has the potential to alter the position of teenagers within society. The most important spaces of citizenship for participants in this research were at the local level. This is not to say that reference was not made to the consideration of a more global arena. For example, global networks of technology were highlighted as an important means of overcoming some of the problems of physical isolation. Furthermore, many participants called for a greater stake in local decision-making. Reflecting back upon the anti-war protests in March 2003, organized by children and teenagers, it is possible to relate these actions to those described by teenagers in this research. These actions indeed both challenge and quash the notion of teenage apathy and should reinforce the need for a broader societal acceptance of teenagers as active citizens in the here and now. Nonetheless, there are also cautionary notes. Whilst many teenagers are actively engaged in different aspects of their communities many barriers remain with regard to teenagers' inclusion in more mainstream political arenas, as we will see in the next chapter.

Chapter 6

Teenagers' exclusion from participation

Introducing teenagers' exclusion

In the late 1960s and early 1970s, advocacy geographers attempted to redefine academic conventions by providing participants with the opportunity to set research agendas (Philo, 1997). The notion of advocacy is also influential today in more contemporary research with children. Matthews *et al.* (2000b), for example, call on researchers to become the link between children and policy-makers. Following the ethos of the advocacy geographers, this study sought to promote the often unheard voices of participants. As part of the dissemination strategy local councillors were sent a short 'findings'[11] report detailing participants' experiences and opinions regarding both the lack of facilities and opportunities for participation as well as examples of teenagers' active involvement. The report also outlined participants' constructive recommendations to the local authority. In a sense the report was intended to be an opportunity for participants to present themselves as active citizens. The first response received from a councillor incited initial laughter, followed by much anger and frustration. Not only had the councillor misinterpreted the findings, but he also reinforced all the feelings of mistrust and disengagement that many teenagers felt towards the council:

> Thank you for your booklet on the activities of teenagers' behaviour, I find it quite informative ... Thankfully we, on the Island, are not subject to any prolonged acts of misbehaviour but I suppose we must always be vigilant, ready to take action when and how it occurs.
> (Response letter from councillor, 15th July 2003)

Whilst chapters 4 and 5 highlighted many positive examples of both teenagers' own acts of citizenship and the ways in which key actors have encouraged and facilitated participants' involvement, much still needs to be done to overcome the kinds of constraints displayed in the councillor's response.

This chapter turns to the exploration of participants' perspectives on the barriers they face to meaningful participation and citizenship. In order to provide a context for their experiences, I begin by examining teenagers' experiences of exclusion in relation to a 'sense of belonging', a lack of facilities and opportunities, and perpetual negative stereotyping. Second, participants' encounters of inclusion and exclusion from local governance are explored. Whilst positive attempts have been made to increase the opportunity for involvement by young teenagers, local decision-makers often use limited methods of gathering opinions and have made uninformed decisions on behalf of teenagers without thorough consultation. Finally, the chapter highlights participants' recommendations to the local authority in order to demonstrate teenagers' competency in the world of mainstream politics.

Constraints to teenagers' citizenship

Drawing upon Lister's (1997a; 1997b) notion that citizenship is exclusive in two dimensions, it is important to examine teenagers' exclusion *from* and exclusion *within* their communities in order to illustrate some of the main constraints to teenagers' citizenship. First, the exploration of participants' sense of belonging in the research locale provides important contextual detail regarding their exclusion. Subsequently, the neglect many participants perceived the local authority has afforded to facilities and services for teenagers are examined. Finally, some of the experiences that participants had of being targeted, stereotyped and, as teenagers, used as scapegoats for local social problems are outlined. The experiences described by participants highlight constraints to teenagers' citizenship in terms of both belonging and opportunities for participation.

A sense of belonging

A sense of belonging has been classified by Jochum *et al.* (2005) as one of the more social elements of active citizenship. France (1998) also argues that 'community life' is significant in fostering young people's identities as citizens. Here, I look at teenagers' sense of belonging as the basis for my later examination of inclusion and exclusion from spaces of citizenship. Participants in the first survey revealed little sense of belonging within their communities. Whilst the majority (63 per cent; n = 425) liked living in their communities, only 34 per cent felt a sense of belonging. Many participants (40 per cent) were either undecided or ambivalent about the question. Whilst a sense of belonging is hard to define these figures are key indicators of teenagers' sense of exclusion from 'mainstream' community life, while later discussions allowed the complexities inherent in the notion of belonging to be explored. For example, Chloe and Katie outlined a geography of (non)belonging on the Island which provided a useful explanation for disparate experiences of inclusion highlighted in the survey:

SUSIE: Where you live do you feel there's like ... um ... a sense of community?
CHLOE/KATIE: No. (Laughs)
CHLOE: I live ... um ... down the road. It's like on the [name] estate ... down [name] road and it's like [estate 2] opposite ... there's no sense of community at all really.
KATIE: Yeah cos I live in [town 1] but there's not that many people living there really compared to [town 2], is there?
CHLOE: ... mostly just old people.
SUSIE: ... do you feel you belong to the community there?
KATIE: Yeah. I sort of do.
CHLOE: I sort of do but not as much as I did when I lived in [town 3] ...
KATIE: Yeah.
CHLOE: ... cos that was like smaller and everybody knew everybody else.

(Group discussion, 3rd July 2002)

Chloe feels that some areas of the Island do have a 'sense of community', where neighbourhoods are close-knit and inclusive (see Halfacree, 1996a; 1996b). A sense of belonging, Relph (1976) suggests, may also have negative connotations. Participants may feel they belong to their communities, whilst simultaneously feeling trapped or isolated. Loki's experiences were rather more negative. As noted previously he lives on a 1950s housing estate ranked within the top 10 per cent of wards in England suffering multiple deprivation (ONS, 2000). Loki encounters many challenges on his estate, particularly between residents and teenagers over the use of space (see plate 15):

LOKI: ... that's where I play football sometimes but I hit the cars and, by accident, ... then people come out and tell us to 'F' off ... Point to my house and say 'that's where I live' and he goes 'bog off up that way then ... a bit more', and that's it.
SUSIE: Mmm, so you get quite a lot of hassle ...
LOKI: Yeah.
SUSIE: ... about what you do and where you go and stuff ...?
LOKI: Yeah. They tell you to move ... go down there. So you go down there and then there's more old people who tell yer to 'F' off. They don't say 'please could you go', they say 'Fuck off'.

(Group discussion, 3rd July 2002)

Loki furthers discussion of his sense of exclusion by highlighting some of the encounters that his friends have had in local spaces:

LOKI: Oh. It's what the old people are like ... it's like you're sat there kicking a football around like that ... you sitting there kicking a football to each other yeah. They come up to yer 'there's a perfectly good field down there'. There's smashed glass bottles, er, you know, stuff like that ...

SUSIE: Yeah.

LOKI: There's a boy ... in the forest there and we play manhunt sometimes and he fell over and there was a bag of heroin needles ...

SUSIE: Really!

LOKI: ... and he got stabbed in his hand and he had to have a blood test but there was nothing ...

(Group discussion, 3rd July 2002)

Loki surmised that he and his friends were not welcome in many areas of their communities. Other residents often instructed them to disperse or gather in other areas. Their presence and activities, therefore, were not seen as legitimate uses of the space. This echoes Reay and Lucey's (2000) notion of a 'child-hostile social landscape' (see also Morrow, 2000). The alternative, more hidden, spaces to where participants relocated often presented other problems, which ultimately led to further exclusion. Reay and Lucey's (2000) exploration of children's lives in inner-city council estates highlights the stigma felt by many residents. Much of Loki's dialogue upholds the sentiment that teenagers are viewed as 'trouble' or threatening. This inherently affected Loki's sense of belonging. He did, however, take some pride in discussing the trouble he had been in. This reflection on Loki's personal narrative highlights how teenagers can reinforce such negative stereotypes.

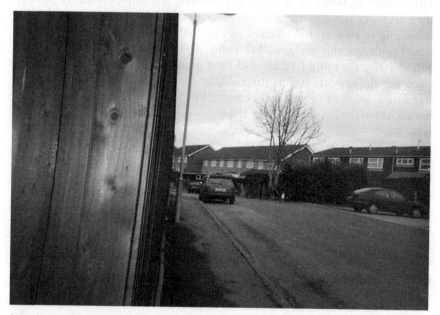

Plate 15 Not belonging, photographed by Loki

Whether Loki's actions contribute to, or are a result of, stereotyped representations of youth, however, is questionable.

A lack of belonging was not always easy to define. Gumdrop, for example, was adamant that there was no sense of community in her local area but could not express her feelings beyond conjecture. Moreover, an individual sense of belonging or a collective sense of community, whether experienced positively or negatively, may not always be interpreted in the same way. Bob struggled to pinpoint why he did feel a sense of belonging. This is somewhat challenging as he was relatively new to the area and had few friends there. Whilst this did not appear of consequence to Bob's sense of belonging, it did matter to Rammstein Nut. She felt that the lack of community in her local area was borne out of tensions between adults and children. Rammstein Nut resides in an isolated hamlet with few children and teenagers:

SUSIE: Is there much of a community down there?
RAMMSTEIN NUT: Um, not really. Do you mean like how many people ... and all bonding together ...
SUSIE: Yeah, yeah.
RAMMSTEIN NUT: ... and stuff like that? No there's just like mainly old people and stuff. We don't sort of ... they're all like stuck up and stuff, and, you know, they don't really like children around.

(Individual interview, 2nd July 2002)

The divided response to a sense of belonging is complex and, as Massey suggests there is 'no single sense of place that everyone shares' (1993: 60). Belonging is an essential element of citizenship, and whilst more conventional understandings regard belonging as significant at the level of the nation-state, the more flexible and fluid approaches outlined in chapter 2 recognize the importance of citizenship at the local level. Moreover, understanding a sense of belonging is essential to feminist conceptualizations of the exclusionary nature of citizenship.

Neglected teenagers

One notable way in which the majority of participants felt a lack of belonging or exclusion from community life was through poor provision of facilities and services. In the first questionnaire, 75 per cent (n = 425) felt there was not enough to do where they lived. Furthermore, 89 per cent specifically called for more facilities for children and teenagers. One adult participant on the iwight web forum felt that the local authority was not placing enough emphasis on the needs of younger people:

It seems that the whole aim of the council is to look after the interests of older/elderly citizens and forget about the youngsters, so long as the youngsters are swept away during Cowes Week [large international yachting festival] when all the rich visitors come, nobody knows any different. It even seems the council are trying to stop legitimate sports. I hear skateboarding is now being banned from roads if performed 'dangerously'. I'd love to know how 'dangerous' is going to be defined! I'd also like to see what the teenagers who used to go skateboarding will do now? Although I can probably guess! How are the youth supposed to get any experiences of 'life' at all when all the council's resources are aimed almost completely at the elderly population?

(Entry on iwight web forum, 12th February 2003)

Many participants felt their attitudes towards the provision of facilities on the Island had changed as they had got older. Several looked back with nostalgia at the plethora of activities available to younger children. Several commented that, as young children, they were happy with simple activities, such as playing in the garden. As teenagers, with greater spatial freedoms, many stated the need for more facilities away from the home:

SUSIE: Have you kinda changed your mind a lot about living on the Island, whether you like it or not, as you've got older?
BOB STEVENS: Yeah.
AGNUZ: Yeah cos when I was younger there was a beach ... just played in the garden. When you're older you like go out and there's not much to do.

(Group discussion, 3rd July 2002)

Kat also lives in a remote village. She specifically draws attention to the only facility in the vicinity, the local shop (see plates 16 and 17).

A lack of public transport and independent mobility were predominant issues. Whilst existing facilities were acknowledged, many felt that there was not enough to do during bad weather or in the evenings:

If I could change where I live I would make more things for young people to do – youth club open more and at the weekend ... I would make more places indoors for young people e.g. cafes aimed at young people ... I would make more open spaces – for recreation.

(Extracts from Gumdrop's diary)

In part, this seasonal and nocturnal problem is related to the Island's economic base. Centred upon tourism, many recreational facilities close in the winter. It is common for teenagers to feel that such facilities cater only for tourists. Such feelings foster resentment and frustration as local decision-makers are seen to be neglecting the needs of teenagers. Moreover, many participants felt that existing facilities were too expensive (see also Morrow, 2003) and inaccessible:

Yeah I think ... I think you've got cases like the cinema and ice skating and stuff but that's like really expensive to get over there for me and it's expensive when you get there as well.

(Discussion with Funda, 2nd July 2002)

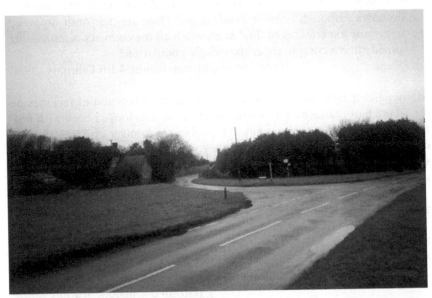

Plate 16 Nothing to do, photographed by Kat

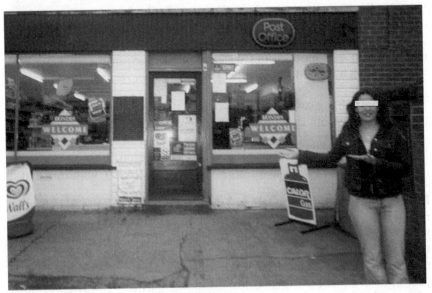

Plate 17 Nowhere to go, photographed by Kat

Some participants were particularly frustrated by the closure of several teenage-orientated facilities. Katie not only states that many facilities focus on the needs of young children but that existing facilities, for example youth clubs, have closed, leaving many teenagers with little to do (see plate 18):

> Um ... (Laughs) that's the town hall. It used to be ... it used to be ... er ... a youth club there but it's ... it's like gone ... gone now ... but it was for like six-year-olds stuff. So there's not much for our age now.
>
> (Group discussion, 3rd July 2002)

Such measures show little respect for teenagers' status or belonging within society, and by no means suggest that teenagers are seen as active and equal citizens. In this scenario teenagers are again situated as 'outsiders'. Their own views and needs do not directly equate to votes, in the same way that perhaps the requirements of younger children might through the voices or votes of their parents. On the Island this is not necessarily the case as facilities for young children are also relatively poor. Only 3 per cent of playgrounds, for example, reach expected performance targets (iwight, 2002).

Loki and Bob Stevens highlight their frustration and confusion at being excluded from local youth clubs. Aged 13 and 14 respectively, they are viewed by some youth clubs as 'too old' to attend:

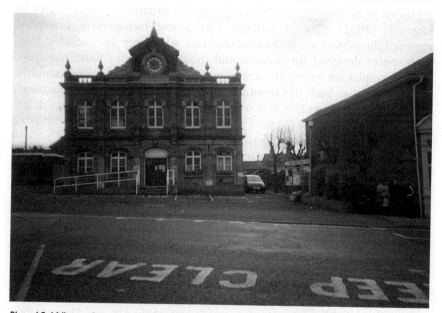

Plate 18 Where the youth club used to be, photographed by Katie

SUSIE: Do you go to youth clubs or anything?

BOB STEVENS: I used to but then I got too old.

LOKI: Yeah they won't let us in.

SUSIE: Really?

LOKI: They say we're too old.

SUSIE: What age is youth club then?

LOKI: It's like ... for year eights [aged approximately 12].

BOB STEVENS: Year eights.

LOKI: They say it's for year eights and that ... The one in [town] they hold it in the thingy ... it's like they won't let us in for it yeah so we just wait outside and they say 'go away or we'll phone the police' and we just like sitting there ... so we've got to go away and if you don't they do actually phone the police.

BOB STEVENS: Can I just say something about the youth club thing?

SUSIE: Yeah sure.

BOB STEVENS: We're still actually youth if you think about it. So why would they want to call the police?

(Group discussion, 3rd July 2002)

Loki and Bob Stevens' experiences demonstrate the challenges that are embodied in the period between childhood, youth and adulthood. They do not 'fit' into any of these categories and are not only excluded from the youth club but criminalized for inhabiting the space. Within the broader context of Loki's narrative some of his actions may, in part, have led to his exclusion or criminalization. Nevertheless, this situation echoes research by Chrisafis (2002) who, in dialogue with young teenagers in Liverpool, reported the neglect many 14-year-olds face when they are excluded from both spaces designed for children and those catering for older teenagers. Such examples underline the continuous juxtaposition between children and teenagers as both threatening and in need of protection (Williamson, 2002). In response to this deficit in facilities the Kids' Club Network are currently pioneering the 'Make Space' scheme, which will provide valuable places for young teenagers to socialise after school (Barton, 2002).

The lack of, and exclusion from, facilities and services on the Island often led to a sense of frustration and lack of power within the community. The results from an online poll conducted on the Island in 2003 suggested that a significant proportion (42 per cent; n = 125) of voters believed that a lack of facilities for teenagers resulted in young people behaving badly. Although this poll is likely to be a reflection of the thoughts of the most vocal members of the Island, who regularly contribute to the iwight web forum, it nevertheless highlights the nexus constructed between 'teenagers' and 'trouble'. Moreover, it is hardly surprising that many teenagers feel 'out of place' or excluded from public space with increasing numbers of 'children-free villages' (Khan, 2003) and curfew zones in areas of the UK (see Davis, 1990;

Travis, 2000; Burrell, 2001; Mendick, 2002; Willow, 2004). Little recognition has been given to the effects of such moves on teenagers' emerging sense of themselves as citizens.

Targeted teenagers

The final major constraint to teenagers' citizenship was participants' experiences of stereotyping and scapegoating. One participant described feeling uncomfortable everywhere she went because of the way in which young people are treated:

> We get shouted at wherever we go! So everywhere.
>
> (Female, aged 14)

The gathering of groups of teenagers is often seen as a criminal threat and demonized (Salvadori, 2001; Kraack and Kenway, 2002). Past research has suggested that teenagers are often blamed for deviant behaviour, and are warranted little status as moral agents in many spheres of society (Mayall, 2000). Loki, rather over-zealously at times, documented the trouble he had been in with various authorities. Indeed he made reference to the 1995 film *Mallrats*, where two teenagers spend their days hanging out in a shopping centre causing trouble. It must, therefore, be remembered that to acknowledge teenagers as competent social actors is also to accept that the actions of some may not always be positive for others. Indeed, some groups of (older) teenagers were regarded as threatening by the participants themselves:

> Out of school I don't feel comfortable walking down ... oh ... what ... I can't remember what the street was but there's this street that ... um ... all these teenagers hang out in that um ... I don't feel comfortable walking down cos they just yell abuse at everyone that walks past and everything ... you just get shouted at all the time by everyone that's your age ... they don't actually know you but they just look at what you're wearing and make a judgement of you.
>
> (Individual interview with Bob, 4th July 2002)

> Wherever older people are – sometimes in the park or along the road.
>
> (Female, aged 13)

> Felt intimidated outside youth club – where older kids hang around – make remarks ... Older kids don't show younger people respect, think they can push us around.
>
> (Extract from Gumdrop's diary)

Respect and fear of being bullied by other teenagers made several participants uncomfortable on a regular basis as the threatening parties hung out in the same spaces. Janna draws attention to the bus stop at the end of her road (see plate 19):

JANNA: There's a bus stop. It's like ... it's changed a bit now but it's somewhere a lot of people just my age hang around and smoke.
SUSIE: Yeah.
JANNA: ... and often, often you feel quite intimidated by ... round the corner, even though I know them ... you know that there's always somebody saying something about you or pointing something out about you ... and I don't really like going past there very much when there's big crowds around it ... bit uneasy there.

(Individual interview, 5th July 2002)

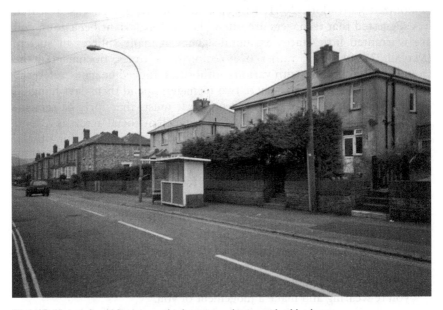

Plate 19 Uncomfortable spaces, the bus stop, photographed by Janna

Whilst many participants hung around in groups of friends, several also felt the presence of gangs was particularly significant in fostering a sense of discomfort or lack of belonging in public spaces. Rammstein Nut discussed this:

RAMMSTEIN NUT: Yeah I feel uncomfortable where there's like lots of older people ... like gangs that I don't know like ...
SUSIE: Yeah.

RAMMSTEIN NUT: ... you know like sort of town people in big groups. Like I was in McDonald's the other day and there was this massive fight and apparently this girl just came out of prison, and another girl and she was just bleeding all over the floor ...

SUSIE: Mmm.

RAMMSTEIN NUT: ... and I felt ... cos it was just horrible. I don't really ... I'm a bit. I don't know I'm not antisocial it's just I don't like people I don't know sort of hanging ... around. I feel uncomfortable around them.

(Individual interview, 2nd July 2002)

Several teenagers devised alternative routes in their communities in order to avoid spaces in which they felt uncomfortable. This echoes feminist writings relating to women's coping strategies in public space. For example, one girl in the survey described how all the local gangs gathered outside the chip shop in her local town. Chloe noted that she avoided Marks and Spencer because of the type of people who hang out there, whilst Kendal opted not to go near his local green as other teenagers smoked there. Several participants also noted experiences of threatening adults. These participants, therefore, are constructing certain types of behaviour in their local spaces as 'other'. As Sibley (1999) suggests, through his psycho-analytical approach to 'sameness' and 'difference', individuals both internalize notions of other(s) as 'good' or 'bad' whilst projecting images of pleasure and anxiety. As a result, individuals construct boundaries around themselves, defining people and places that are not like them as 'other'. Not only are the participants in my research excluding themselves from such spaces but they are also displaying their norms and values in relation to what is constructed as (in)appropriate or threatening behaviour within those arenas.

Despite the complexity of threatening behaviour it was not uncommon for participants to be unjustifiably accused of 'deviant' acts and monitored by local authorities. The story from Loki, Agnuz and Bob Stevens is one of struggle: struggle against prejudice. Loki tells of his struggle to stay out of trouble on his deprived council estate whilst being faced with regular blame for anti-social behaviour:

LOKI: I've got the typical routine of an old person 'I KNOW YOUR PARENTS!'

SUSIE: (Laughs)

LOKI: 'Who are they are then?' 'I know them.' 'Don't get lippy with me boy.' 'What?' 'Don't answer me back. Do you want some of this (fist)? I'll chase you I will.' (in a shrill voice)

SUSIE: Do you ... do you ever get moved on from where you hang out?

BOB STEVENS: Sometimes.

AGNUZ: Yeah.

LOKI: Mmm.

SUSIE: Who ... who by?

LOKI: Police. Old people mostly.

SUSIE: Do they tell you why you shouldn't be there?

LOKI: No. They go 'move on, move out the way. You're causing trouble' or we're loitering ...

AGNUZ: Cos you're thinking you're not doing anything wrong and they just chuck you out cos down [supermarket] we're just sitting on the wall there eating crisps and stuff and they like come out and go stop skating there ... and we didn't even have skateboards with us! And they went and phoned the police.

(Group discussion, 3rd July 2002)

Loki and Agnuz also described the surveillance that teenagers face in private, commercial spaces. In particular they discussed their experiences in a large music store where they felt their presence was seen as suspicious or potentially criminal. Shopping centres are significant social sites for many teenagers (Matthews *et al.*, 2000a; White and Sutton, 2001). Loki and Agnuz's encounters reflect the work of Sibley (1995), who examined spaces of exclusion within shopping centres. He details a documentary, the subtext of which highlighted the surveillance and control of 'undesirables', mainly teenagers, who did not 'fit in' to the family-orientated image of the shopping centre. This image is often sanitized and exclusive (White and Sutton, 2001). This situation not only demonstrates the lack of trust many teenagers feel adults afford them (see also Morrow, 2000; 2003) but also highlights the difficulties in regarding consumerism as an arena in which young people have greater access to citizenship (Stuart, 2000; Valentine, 2000).

Discussions with Loki, Bob Stevens and Agnuz revealed an explicit geography of surveillance, regulation and conflict (Weller, 2003). They referred to specific spaces where their presence, often because of their age, was not welcomed or tolerated:

There's tons of big fields. We go and play manhunt in 'em, but the old people, I think it's the farmers probably all walk their dogs through and they tell us to clear off. They tell us to 'F' off and 'go away you little fuckers' ... cos you run along the footpaths and they come running off the fields ... we don't smash up the crops or nothing. We just find tracks and jump in and hide.

(Group discussion, 3rd July 2002)

Hanging out within public spaces was, however, often highly regulated. Such control of what was perceived to be dangerous or 'deviant' behaviour was often centred upon particular pursuits, such as skateboarding:

KENDAL: ... when you're skating on the street and stuff cos it's the sort of place you get told off by the police and that's ... take your name down and stuff.

SUSIE: Yeah.

KENDAL: And that's annoying. Even though there's a skate park there's other bits in [town] that are like good for skateboarding ... and the cops don't like it so you get told off sometimes then.

SUSIE: Is there anything they can do about it?

KENDAL: Yeah sometimes if they give you three or four warnings and like they can take your board off you ...

SUSIE: Really?

KENDAL: ... yeah, and like confiscate it and you can't get it back. They give you the warning. Even if you're like skating down to the skate park they'll still stop you, take your name down. I've been stopped a couple of times.

(Group discussion, 4th July 2002)

'Deviant' behaviour has been targeted on the Island. CCTV has been installed on local public transport to prevent vandalism (IWCP, 2002a). The local authority also developed a scheme which placed 'naughty' children and teenagers on a separate and very distinct pink school bus. One participant in the iwight web forum discussion expressed her disgust at the scheme:

As a children's rights officer I am absolutely appalled by the Pink Peril bus initiative. You should be ashamed of yourselves. How on earth do you expect to engender a sense of responsibility, community and self-worth in kids who are having problems with school by humiliating them in public? ... It will foster an even greater sense of exclusion in kids who think that education isn't for them ... We complain about children's behaviour and label them a social nuisance but we are often the cause of that behaviour through not listening to them, not involving them and not meeting their needs. If I walked up to a shop which had a notice in its window which read 'no more than two women in this shop at one time', how would I feel? If 'reasonable chastisement' were a legal defence for a man to beat me without being punished, how would I feel? How would you feel?

(iwight web forum, VI Lenin)

VI Lenin's posting on the web-board draws attention to a number of issues relating to teenagers' lack of status as citizens. Indeed, the contributor suggests that exclusion of this nature could have a detrimental impact upon many of the elements associated with the citizenship curriculum, such as fostering a sense of responsibility. On the web forum and in other local media this view was, however, in the minority. Many advocated the scheme as a viable solution to the perceived 'youth problem'. Central to the notion of 'youth as threatening' is the dichotomy between 'young' and 'old'. Many participants felt that ageism was rife on the Island and as a result believed their activities and presence were highly regulated and monitored. Many also felt they had become scapegoats for trouble and crime, yet at the same time several participants constructed their own stereotypes of older people as intolerant:

> The Island youth don't feel like they belong because of the ageist atti-tudes that are so prominent. They are looked upon as troublemakers before anything has been done so that the elderly population thinks things are under control and safe for their little retirement village.
>
> (iwight web forum, Carl)

The correlation between teenagers and troublemaking has to end in order to appreciate teenagers not as agents of deviancy but as active contributors to their communities (Roche, 1999; Weller, 2003). This is particularly sig-nificant as age-based stereotypes result in teenagers believing they are of lower status and have fewer rights, as one participant argues:

> Everyone thinks that all teenagers are trouble makers so we get less rights.
>
> (Female, aged 14)

Many teenagers felt marginalized and left out of their communities, primar-ily because of their embodiment as young. Their activities and interests are seen to be in conflict with the rest of the community and, as a result, younger people often feel undervalued. The resentment incited by the lack of belonging experienced by many teenagers renders active participation and involvement in the community problematic. As detailed in chapter 5, feelings of exclusion and a lack of rights may motivate a number of teenagers to bring about change by other means, although in the main such exclusion is likely to deter many from taking on social responsibilities (France, 1998). Nonetheless, teenagers do have some experiences of being listened to and heard by local decision-makers.

Being heard in the community

Having outlined the barriers to participants' sense of belonging the follow-ing section of this chapter moves on to explore teenagers' encounters of inclusion within and exclusion from local governance by highlighting the extent to which participants felt listened to and, more importantly, *heard* by local decision-makers.

Being listened to

In 2002 the charity Childline commissioned the study *Are Young People Being Heard?* (RBA, 2002). Only one-third (n = 1387) of participants rated national or local government as 'good' at listening to the needs of children and young people. For those aged 11–16, not being listened to conjured up feelings of both anger and also acceptance that it was the 'norm' not to be listened to. Several measures have, however, been taken by local government to involve teenagers in decision-making (JRF, 2002; Freeman *et al.*, 2003). Indeed, global ventures such as the UNCRC and Agenda 21[12] encourage the incorporation of children and young people in decision-making (Freeman, 1999; Chawla, 2001; Freeman *et al.*, 2003). The 2003 Government Green Paper *Every Child Matters* also states that decision-makers should provide children and teenagers with opportunities for participation (DfES, 2003). Nevertheless, one-fifth of local authorities in the UK do not have any systems of consultation in place to listen to children and teenagers (Monahan, 2002). In the first questionnaire in this study 81 per cent (n = 425) stated that they had *never* been asked their opinion on a local issue(s). Of the 19 per cent (n = 425) of participants who had been consulted, the matters discussed included ideas for improving communities, crime and disorder, traffic and transport, and the development of skate parks.

When positive action does occur, it is often in the form of a youth forum or parliament (see Matthews and Limb, 1998; Probert, 2001; JRF, 2002). Forums and parliaments are significant arenas for teenagers to engage not only in citizenship but in dialogue with local decision-makers (Weller, 2003). On the Island, several opportunities for participation exist. A youth council is being developed to work alongside local government (IWCP, 2002b). On a smaller scale some villages have founded youth forums, and consultation has been undertaken on a variety of activity-based issues, such as the building of skate parks. A youth parliament, 'Wight2BHeard', has also been created, which annually involves around 160 children and teenagers and 40 adults including the MP and local councillors (Wight Insight, 2001; Rutland, 2002). In this parliament delegates participate in voting, questionnaire completion and general debates on Island-based issues. For some, the structure of the parliament has brought about very real and positive outcomes, as one of the organisers highlighted (Weller, 2003):

> The event actually came about from a conference [youth parliament] I organized ... where we had a lot of senior figures on the Island ... and a young lady stood up and said 'can Wight Leisure organize something for young people on the Island as part of the festival?' and that's how this came about ... Umm ... and ... you know, all credit to her for doing

that because if she hadn't have done that and this young lady hadn't have spoken out the event last night wouldn't have happened and, of course, it did and it WAS a great success ...

(Caller, male, adult on the local radio phone-in, 6th June 2002)

One participant requested more events be organized for children and teenagers under 18. The youth parliament responded with a dance night. The parliament does, however, only include a minute proportion of children and teenagers on the Island (0.5 per cent). Results from the first questionnaire suggested that only 12 per cent (n = 425) of respondents had been involved in any form of youth forum or council. Of those, 55 per cent (n = 54) felt the points that they raised had been considered seriously. Whilst delegates represent other local teenagers, most participants in this research were both unaware of the existence of the local youth parliament and had not been invited to participate (Morrow, 2003; Weller, 2003), as Chloe and Katie discuss:

SUSIE: It's called 'Wight2BHeard' youth parliament. Did you hear anything about that?
KATIE: No.
CHLOE: That's the first time I've ever heard about it.
SUSIE: Oh that's interesting. That's a shame, isn't it? Do you think you'd like to join in with something like that? Is it something you'd want to do?
CHLOE: I think if the school was asked um ... quite a majority of people would go ...
KATIE: Mmm.
CHLOE: ... cos people are fed up with not having much to do here.

(Group discussion, 3rd July 2002)

Access to such spaces of citizenship is fundamental to the creation of inclusive arenas for participation. Many teenagers believed it was good ideological practice, with several keen to be involved if they felt they would be able to discuss issues relevant to their lives. Nevertheless, it did not appear to have impacted upon many of the participants in this research to date. Indeed, several were sceptical that it would have any real effect:

It can't be that effective cos nothing ever changes. I don't actually think they'd listen. I think they'd just make out as if they're listening but not actually do anything about it.

(Discussion with Nikki, 2nd July 2002)

This situation mirrors Smith et al.'s (2002) observations that those who are already disenfranchised often question the worth of youth-specific forums.

Several participants had, however, benefited from smaller scale forms of participation such as village forums, as Kat outlines:

KAT: We've got this other place where we go up in a little church room and we're discussing whether we should have a skate park or not. We've got our own little council thing ...
SUSIE: What like a youth council?
KAT: Yeah.

(Group discussion, 4th July 2002)

As detailed in chapter 5, Kat had participated in the 'busie' project within her relatively isolated village, which eventually led to the development of a youth forum. It is important, though, to highlight at this stage the significance of participation and inclusion at the micro-level. Smaller scale forums not only have the potential to include more teenagers but also afford participants the opportunity to discuss some of their most pressing everyday needs and issues. Gumdrop noted how she felt listened to at youth club by a visitor:

Man came to speak to us about a 'one-stop' shop – information centre for young people – listened to our opinions.

(Extract from Gumdrop's diary)

Local decision-makers or 'professionals', as Freeman *et al.* (2003) suggest, play a fundamental role in shaping teenagers' opportunities for citizenship. Many participants (38 per cent; n = 367) felt that the local council made most of the important decisions regarding their communities. Respondents also suggested parish councils (8 per cent) and adults/old people (7 per cent) influenced local decision-making. Other alternatives included the community, the MP, local churches and the government. Just over one-quarter (26 per cent) stated that they did not know who determined the outcome of local issues. Moreover, there was a great deal of antipathy towards the local council. Several teenagers described local decision-makers in ways that suggested they were not in tune with the needs of children and teenagers:

The old fogies councillors who ain't got a clue what they're on about.
(Male, aged 13)

Old, fat, rich men who don't care what kids think [council].
(Male, aged 15)

I think if they [those who make important decisions] know a child has wrote or phoned they'll scrap the issue or say they're busy or something.
(Male, aged 13)

Freeman *et al.* (2003) suggest that, whilst local authorities have endeav-
oured to include teenagers in decision-making, for a variety of motivations,
the approach(es) used are often inappropriate. This 'imposed agenda' finds
professionals attempting to incorporate young people into systems which
are not accustomed to working with them. These systems are often hierarchical, use traditional methods of consultation such as questionnaires, and
work within electoral time periods. What is most significant, however, is
that the majority of participants had not had *any* opportunities to contribute to local decision-making. Nikki stated that her participation in this
research was the only time she had been asked her opinion on local issues:

> It's the only time we've ever been listened to and it's on tape!
>
> (Group discussion, 2nd July 2002)

For the teenagers in this research the 'consultation fatigue' that many
researchers (Davies and Marken, 2000) fear was obviously not an issue.
Moreover, merely listening to teenagers' voices is not sufficient and is in
danger of becoming less than tokenistic. Actually *hearing* teenagers' voices
is thus important.

Being heard

For many participants frustration resulted from both a feeling of not being
consulted and being excluded from political institutions (see also Wyn and
White, 1997). Participation is constructed as an 'adult' activity, carried out
in adult institutions. Children and teenagers are often only afforded the status of 'taking part' (Wellard *et al.*, 1997), as full participation is frequently
regarded as a threat to adult autonomy. As Willow argues:

> To be respected as real people, children have to shed their childhood
> skin and become adults.
>
> (2004: 28)

The solutions that authorities provide to what they perceive as the key
issues or problems are also often misguided:

> SUSIE: Do you like living here?
> JANNA: Err ... I like ... I like some of it ... I mean I like the ... umm ...
> feel of the Island. It's very like nice place to live ... if you're not my age,
> because there's nothing to do. I mean people say 'oh yeah there's a skate
> park' blah, blah, blah but it isn't actually that good and it ... You could
> have done with children planning it instead of someone that doesn't
> actually know anything about skating.
>
> (Individual interview, 5th July 2002)

Several participants discussed the use of questionnaires by local decision-makers to gauge teenagers' views (Morrow, 2003; Weller, 2003). Whilst this was seen as a positive step towards incorporating teenagers into decision-making processes, the use of questionnaires limited the extent to which participants could elaborate upon their opinions and ideas:

CHLOE: I've done like questionnaires before but never been like ... asked like my actual ... true opinions ...

SUSIE: So when you did the questionnaire did you feel it was written to get like the answers they wanted?

CHLOE: Yeah.

SUSIE: Did you feel that what ... what you wrote was ever listened to? Did they ever do anything about [it]?

CHLOE: No ...

(Group discussion, 3rd July 2002)

Consultation, therefore, was seen as ineffective and tokenistic and, perhaps more fundamentally, seldom resulted in any real action:

KITTY SANDORAL: I've done like a couple of surveys and stuff ... and people like drop things through your door and stuff like that. And I've done ... um ... like through school and stuff people just ask you your opinion on things.

SUSIE: Do you think your opinion has ever been listened to?

KITTY SANDORAL: No (Laughs) they listen to you but they don't actually do anything about it. Do you know what I mean? It was a waste of time. I mean they come in and ask you something and then they just leave it at that. That's all that they do and they don't do anything about it ... follow it up or anything.

SUSIE: So is there anyone in particular you think who's kind of ignored you?

KITTY SANDORAL: I did a survey for the council asking about what they... if we could have anything new in [town] what would they want and they didn't do anything I don't think. They just ... they did the survey I think and ... um ... I handed it in and all that stuff, and I didn't get any reply or anything and they didn't follow anything through.

(Group discussion, 2nd July 2002)

Whilst the opportunities designed to embrace teenagers in local decision-making go some way to develop inclusive spaces of citizenship, these arenas soon become *frustrating spaces of citizenship* if they do not allow participants fully to express their ideas and opinions. Furthermore, once listened to, participants were annoyed at the lack of solutions or feedback on the outcomes of the consultation. Arguably, this form of consultation is not truly participatory and such an approach can heighten cynicism and frustration (Freeman *et al.*, 2003). Many felt their views had just been ignored by authorities who provided misplaced solutions to what they perceived to be the important issues (Matthews, Limb and Taylor, 1999; Weller, 2003). This frequently led to a great deal of resentment from teenagers who felt they were not being taken seriously (O'Toole, 2003), as one mother on the iwight web forum argues:

> You are joking, they don't even get treated with respect in Mcdonalds! What chance have they of being heard!
>> (iwight web forum, mother of two boys, 4th March 2003)

The poignant message that many teenagers wished to express to local decision-makers was that it was not only important to listen to their views and needs, but to create ways in which children and teenagers could actively participate in decisions which affect their lives and the wider community. This is central to fostering a sense of citizenship and empowering young people:

> One point which has been made a couple of times is the decision making power that the Island's youth possess, or rather the lack of. The power to make decisions is perhaps something which the Island's youth need, to give them a sense of responsibility and respect. The youth see the council as the big bad; the authority that doesn't listen. Currently the only power the youth have is to suggest and complain to the council, they have no direct power or influence over changes to the Island. What I suggest is that the Island's younger generation is given the responsibility to make decisions. They should be encouraged to come along to local council meetings to air their views, and they must be listened to. The Island's current demographic is weighed down very much by the elderly, and youth are seen by many as inferior, but we must remember this is their Island too! Let's encourage the voices of tomorrow to help shape this Island into a place they are proud of, not one they are resentful of.
>> (iwight web forum, John, 26th March 2003)

As John's entry on the iwight web forum argues, providing teenagers with opportunities to participate, if they so wish, is fundamental to the prevention of resentment and disillusionment between teenagers and local (adult) decision-makers. Many teenagers also felt stereotyped by local decision-makers who responded to what they perceived to be the needs of teenagers. The most common example was skate parks. Many felt that these had been constructed in response to a lack of facilities for teenagers without recognizing that young people are a diverse social group with many different needs and interests, as Kitty Sandoral and Gumdrop emphasize:

KITTY SANDORAL: ... it's like adults design all these things but they don't really know what we want cos ...

GUMDROP: ... they think every single person under 16 wants to go to skate parks ... Yeah everybody wants to go to skate parks. Like not everybody's into skating.

(Group discussion, 2nd July 2002)

It is apparent that the underlying philosophies of the NSSC have not, in the main, reached policy and practice at the local level.

Participants in this research described not only the denial of children and teenagers as political and social actors, but also the homogenization of young people as a social group. Many participants believed that it was essential to involve children and teenagers in planning processes in order to develop facilities and services which met *their* needs. Several participants called for inclusion in more mainstream political decision-making. This opposes the spatial separation of teenagers' citizenship and calls into question the effectiveness of distinct youth forums and parliaments. Many called for the age at which citizens can participate in elections to be lowered, as Katie stated in her diary:

I think voting should drop to the age of 15.

(Extract from Katie's diary)

Several participants also both challenged the notion of teenage apathy as well as providing suggestions for increasing teenagers' contributions to their communities. Other participants, however, remained sceptical:

SUSIE: Yeah. Would you vote if you could?

FUNDA: I don't think I would. It doesn't interest me ... to be honest ...

NIKKI: It doesn't interest me either. Once they are elected ... once there is someone elected I don't think they really do anything. I think it's pointless.

FUNDA: They just have a higher power and get more money for doing nothing really and get all the credit for everything.

(Group discussion, 2nd July 2002)

Local decision-makers work within wider societal discourses which construct children and teenagers as citizens-in-the-making. Some work has however been done to improve the decision-making opportunities presented to teenagers:

The way forward is to ensure that this goodwill is harnessed and directed towards more effective and meaningful participation. It may be, that rather than arguing for increasing or better participation for young people in the existing local government system perhaps we should be arguing for a total review of how the system operates.

(Freeman *et al.*, 2003: 67)

Nevertheless, Williamson (2002) argues that policies in relation to, for example, children's rights, education and social welfare fail to prioritize the needs of children and teenagers. Instead, policies are directed towards teenagers' perceived needs or the requirements of their parents. Ultimately, they suggest, within this (mainstream) realm young people have little political agency.

Talking as competent citizens

The final section of this chapter is concerned with challenging the notion of teenage apathy by highlighting some of the recommendations participants put forward to the local authority in terms of both the changes they would like to see implemented in the local area and the importance of recognizing their expertise. It concludes with a discussion on participants' perceptions of their status within society in terms of the rights they are afforded.

Challenging apathy

Despite government concerns over youth apathy, 72 per cent (n = 425) of respondents in the second survey desired opportunities to voice their opinions, echoing Freeman *et al.*'s (2003) research in New Zealand. Chloe and Katie are an example of this view:

KATIE: I think like more participation between the community and more opinions and stuff about what needs to be done ...
CHLOE: Yeah. We need to be asked our opinions on things.

(Group discussion, 3rd July 2002)

Participants involved in in-depth elements of this research demonstrated varying degrees of interest in community life. For some, this concerned very specific, youth-centred facilities such as skate parks or youth clubs, whilst for others a more holistic approach to participation was required on the part of local decision-makers. When participants were asked what they would change about where they live, most called for more facilities. In particular, many requested more amenities for both younger and older people, cheaper facilities, more places to socialize, and more skate parks. Other suggestions included 'less traffic', 'safety', 'less boredom', 'less old people' and 'more say over what happens'. Kaz and Kimbo reinforced questionnaire respondents' suggestions by calling for more activities and events:

SUSIE: OK. If you could like suggest one thing that would make your community better what would it be?

KIMBO: More things to do.

KAZ: Yeah.

SUSIE: Any things in particular?

KAZ: Like the swimming pool and stuff.

SUSIE: Yeah, yeah.

KIMBO: Lots of things for little kids to do, like going to theme parks and stuff and teenagers.

KAZ: And I think they should hold more concerts on the Island like say down [town] rec ... hold one there but I can't see they've ever thought of that.

(Group discussion, 4th July 2002)

More specific requests from one group of teenagers included an indoor skate park so that their interest could be pursued all year round:

What I would basically like/love to see would be an indoor skate park with a 'chill out' room which you could sit in and have a rest after skating. In this room you could purchase (cheap) food and drinks and chat with mates.

(Extract from Duey's diary)

Some participants wished to see changes which would be more inclusive, and would cater for the neglected needs of younger people more generally:

SUSIE: And what kind of um ... facilities would you like to see on the Island?

JANNA: Something for ... there's a lot of young people on the Island and even though they say it's becoming an old place but people have to grow up to be old and there's a lot of people still growing up ...

SUSIE: Yeah.

JANNA: ... and er ... although the Island's mostly populated by old people there's still a large percent that are ... aren't young ... I mean aren't old and they ... I think they need to be listened to and I dunno ... I couldn't ... I can't really say what would make it better because I don't really know but I think most people just want somewhere to go ... just somewhere to hang out really.

(Individual interview, 5th July 2002)

Again, Janna (above) highlights the age-related boundaries that many teenagers construct around older people, thus themselves reinforcing the dichotomy between childhood and adulthood.

Much discussion revolved around creating not just amenities for teenagers, but facilities which would have positive benefits for the whole

community. Kendal, Tommey and Matt, for example, suggested that building a sports facility encompassing a large hall, badminton and tennis courts
and a 50-metre swimming pool would allow the Island to enter the 'Island
Games', thus bringing revenue for the tourist and transport industries.
Other teenagers called for a large, centrally located, indoor skate park. This
again could be used for national competitions. Both Rammstein Nut and
Chloe also called for wider changes which bring different elements of the
community together. Their vision is for greater social cohesion as
Rammstein Nut highlights:

SUSIE: If you could suggest one thing that would make your community better what ... what would you suggest if you could think of anything?
RAMMSTEIN NUT: Er ... (Pause) something to make the whole community
come together like old people ... youth ... I don't know what but something that would interest all ages really ...
SUSIE: Yeah.
RAMMSTEIN NUT: I'm not sure cos old people normally hate what young people like ...

(Individual interview, 2nd July 2002)

Kat asked for facilities which would improve the reputation of her village:

People vandalise in [village] because there is nothing to do. We need a
park. Otherwise [village] is going to be called a shit tip for ever.

(Extract from Katie's diary)

In contrast to the notion of teenage apathy, many participants in this
research had ideas and visions for improvements in their locales both for
children and teenagers, as well as for the wider community (see also
Morrow, 2003). Thinking through such issues demonstrates what may be
classified as one of the more social elements of active citizenship where individuals think beyond their own needs. The challenges and frustrations
experienced by broader discourses which brand teenagers as troublemakers,
coupled with the lack of suitable and accessible methods of participation in
local decision-making, fostered a feeling of scepticism amongst many
teenagers, leading them to question whether they can ever possess any
power or influence.

Valuing teenagers' expertise

A fundamental shift towards recognizing that teenagers are competent
social and political actors is needed in order to afford young people greater
status as citizens, as Funda and Nikki argue:

FUNDA: Let's say ... let's say on poor places yeah the adults in the school could say 'oh we know this blah, blah, blah' but a child that is actually poor would know more about it than an adult ...

SUSIE: Yeah.

NIKKI: Exactly.

FUNDA: ... and that's the way I see it. A child could ... it just depends what you've been through and I don't think it's fair the way teachers treat us ... or adults for that matter look down on you. Urgh can't stand it!

(Group discussion, 2nd July 2002)

Reflecting upon discussions of young people's competency in chapter 2, it is important to value teenagers as experts on their own needs (Davies and Marken, 2000). Kendal and Matt felt this recognition was fundamental to understanding the needs of teenagers, as well as of the wider community:

KENDAL: Cos if they asked us like what our opinion was as young people then they'd have more of an idea of what to be able to do and build for the people to do ...

SUSIE: Yeah.

KENDAL: ... rather than sort of guessing.

MATT: Then do something about it.

KENDAL: Yeah because sometimes the council just builds skate parks which are no use cos um ... they build them wrong like put the wrong pieces in the wrong places ...

SUSIE: Yeah.

KENDAL: ... so you've got good skate parks but all the bits are in the wrong places and it would be better if they asked children where they wanted the stuff to go.

MATT: Get everyone to join in ... move it and put it where it's actually meant to be.

(Group discussion, 4th July 2002)

Interest within the community involves not only the energy of teenagers but also concerted efforts from decision-makers to devise methods of participation which inspire and motivate children and teenagers. As Putnam argues:

What we need is not civic broccoli – good for you but unappealing – but an updated version of Scouting's ingenious combination of values and fun.

(2000: 406)

But these methods need to incorporate teenagers' rights.

Recognizing teenagers' rights

Although many participants showed an interest in community life, few felt they were afforded many rights as teenagers. In the second survey 23 per cent (n = 172; 33 per cent did not respond) believed that, as a teenagers, they had few or no rights at all:

> Not many – not a child but too young to do adult things.
>> (Unknown respondent)

> We don't have a lot because everybody thinks that all teenagers are trouble makers so we get less rights.
>> (Female, aged 14)

A small proportion (8 per cent) disagreed, stating that they felt they had a lot of rights. In terms of specific rights for teenagers 7 per cent (n = 172) responded by suggesting they had the right to an education, whilst 6 per cent believed they had the right to be respected, and a further 6 per cent stated they had the right to have their opinions listened to:

> Right to education. Right to be treated equally.
>> (Female, aged 14)

> The right to get asked what we think, not just at school.
>> (Female, aged 15)

> The right to our own opinion and beliefs.
>> (Female, aged 15)

> Right to learn, right to be protected. Right to free speech. Right of opinion.
>> (Male, aged 14)

> To enjoy life and not be treated as a horrible teenager but as an adult.
>> (Male, aged 14)

This summary of participants' interests within their communities coupled with their perceived status in terms of rights suggests that many do not feel empowered by formal political institutions to change radically the places in which they live. The extent to which other members of society feel empowered by local politics is also questionable (see Foley and Martin, 2000). Those under the age of sixteen, however, are much less likely to be engaged in conventional civic participation than all other age groups, with the exception of those over seventy-five (Attwood et al., 2003). In 1998 the

Government White Paper *Modern Local Government: In Touch with the People* recognized the need for major changes in participatory systems to (re)engage British citizens (DETR, 1998). Within the context of contemporary local government practice, Sharp (2002) highlights the notion of 'participation management', where participants are often 'chosen' for the views that they are likely to put across. The increasing focus by local government on 'partnership' with particular organizations also adds an element of selection to local participatory systems (Gibbs *et al.*, 2001). Whilst selection may benefit teenage-centred groups in some areas of the UK, such practice is not evident in this research locale. Moreover, young teenagers remain constitutionally excluded from mainstream spaces of citizenship, for example, by their exclusion from voting in local elections.

Fostering teenagers' citizenship

Exclusion from citizenship and political engagement in local decision-making, a lack of suitable facilities and frequent negative stereotypes in local and more global discourses profoundly affected teenagers' feelings of belonging and engagement. Several cited encounters which uphold the notion of 'threatening youth'. Yet whilst the activities of some might pose a threat to others within society, this was not the case for the majority. Nevertheless, such negative stereotypes held important implications for teenagers' sense of worth as citizens. With the exception of some opportunities for participation there was a general air of despondency: a feeling of 'what's the point, no-one will listen anyway'. Here, participants experienced much of what Lister (1997a; 1997b) refers to as exclusion *from* and exclusion *within* citizenship. Not only were the majority of participants excluded from mainstream practices of citizenship by virtue of their age, but many felt that the opportunities available for participation were not *meaningfully* participatory. With a limited stake in their local communities, many felt that they were afforded little status, respect and few or fewer rights. The positioning of participants as young teenagers in the transitional period between childhood, youth and adulthood furthered these tensions. Many felt they simply did not fit in: too old for some activities and too young for others. In these terms many teenagers are not only excluded from local governance within their communities, but from everyday spaces and amenities.

Participants' sense of frustration was often targeted towards local decision-makers. The vast majority of participants had never been consulted over a local issue. Those who had, revealed often misguided consultation, the practices of which used traditional methods not necessarily suited to engaging in consultation with teenagers. Furthermore, many felt that these consultations were meaningless and did not result in any real action.

Local decision-makers play an important role in shaping teenagers' lives. There was, however, much antipathy towards the local government.

The principally age-defined boundaries between teenagers and local decision-makers were mutually defined. Not only did those in power construct boundaries between themselves and teenagers, but many teenagers themselves created their own barriers and stereotypes of 'old, fat, rich men'. It is apparent that many participants wanted to be involved in the political mainstream. It is also clear that the adoption of the principles of the UNCRC or indeed the philosophies of the NSSC would be beneficial to decision-makers' understandings of teenagers' diverse needs and interests. The relatively recent Government Green Paper *Every Child Matters* is a positive step towards achieving this (DfES, 2003). Nevertheless, many participants described frustrating spaces of exclusion, of non-belonging, of not being heard, of superficial consultation, of little status and of stereotypes resulting in much frustration and despondency. In contrast to the local councillor's comments cited at the beginning of this chapter are the wise words of Delfos (2001) who argues that adult modesty is key to the empowerment of children.

At the heart of participants' frustration lies the differential in power and status of (adult) 'professionals' who are generally regarded as full citizens who educate, mould and sometimes dominate young citizens-in-the-making. Many participants in this research demonstrated their competency in terms of thinking through and acting as citizens, showing innovative, creative and sometimes controversial acts of citizenship. If encouraged and supported via meaningful practices of consultation and 'partnership' these acts have the potential to enhance teenagers' status and sense of belonging.

Chapter 7

Alternative understandings of teenagers' citizenship

Introducing alternative understandings

The research detailed in this book proved to be a considerable journey of learning and often surprise, challenging and stretching my own understandings of teenagers' lives and their relationship with citizenship. Following Philo's (2003) work on memories of childhood, I frequently recollected and pondered upon my own experiences and memories of growing up in the case study area. Similarities between many participants' experiences and my own childhood and teenage years were revealed. Nevertheless, and wholly expected, there were also many disparities. I greatly admire those who have been creative in their acts of citizenship and who have challenged ingrained systems in an attempt to change their communities. In addition to the feelings of many participants, I am also frustrated at the continued neglect of teenagers' voices. Following in the footsteps of past and present advocacy geographers, I made attempts to foster constructive connections between the participants and local policy-makers. Encounters with such decision-makers frequently created frustrating spaces of (non)citizenship for me as I felt I had, to some degree, let down my participants. In the quest for socially relevant research, it was often challenging to maintain the notion that 'I can make a difference', or even whether it is within the bounds of the researcher to do so. It is difficult to evaluate the extent to which decision-makers within the local communities (less so within the school) in the case study area acknowledged the findings disseminated to them. The research received interest from the local MP and a number of councillors, some of whom frustratingly misinterpreted the research findings! This was, at times, an uphill struggle, which enhanced my empathy towards the participants.

As chapter 1 detailed, the research was situated within one rural county in England which, as an island, inherently occupied specific local contexts. Other rural, or indeed urban, areas may be situated within different local social, political, economic and cultural circumstances. Broad generalizations were never an objective of the study. Rather, a case study approach was adopted in order to examine teenagers' experiences in a more holistic manner (see Yin, 1989) gathering detail on the minutiae of teenagers' everyday lives both within and outside school. Such an approach revealed their alternative and innovative connections with citizenship. Findings from the study do have broader national and international resonances. The widespread exclusion and stereotyping of teenagers as (a) social group(s), coupled with the neglect of their active engagement with citizenship, is likely to be apparent in other locales, albeit refracted and interpreted in different ways through individual biographies. The case study area exists within national social, political and economic policy contexts. For example, whilst teenagers' experiences of citizenship education are likely to vary from school to school the underlying rationale and the understanding of citizenship employed in the policy development affects teenagers throughout England. On a global level the influence of the international UNCRC and networks of communication and power were also of particular significance. As such, important lessons can be learnt from participants' perspectives that may be echoed nationally and internationally.

In this final chapter I begin by reflecting upon the context and purpose of the research. Subsequently, three key arguments are presented which together place teenagers' alternative understandings and identities as citizens within a broader context concerning teenagers' current status within Western society. The first of these themes relates to teenagers' relationship with citizenship as it is commonly defined within liberal democracies. The spaces of citizenship explored here have differing temporal logics (Weller, 2003). The rhetoric of citizenship education is concerned with developing responsible citizens in the future, whilst examples of teenagers' engagement within the informal school and in the wider community reveal alternative and often unrecognized acts of citizenship taking place in the here-and-now. The second and third themes are, therefore, concerned with citizenship within school and citizenship in the wider community respectively. Importantly, this concluding chapter argues for a shift in the direction of citizenship education discourse and the utilization of wider definitions of citizenship in British policy towards a more cosmopolitan and inclusive understanding. My proposed approach views children and teenagers as citizens in the here-and-now recognizing their acts of engagement in a variety of spheres. Moreover, this approach regards citizenship as a cumulative process in which children, teenagers and adults are viewed as full citizens who, throughout their life, learn, develop and exert different forms of citizenship in different spaces. I, therefore, seek to present some constructive and challenging messages for both policy and practice.

Re-contextualizing the study

The overriding aim of the research was to examine teenagers' perspectives on and experiences of citizenship in a number of settings. As chapter 1 detailed, the rationale for focusing upon the lives of young teenagers emerged out of three important research and policy contexts. First, and as some other authors have documented (see, for example, Valentine, 2003), young teenagers are the neglected 'others' of research with children and young people. Young teenagers' experiences are particularly important to explore within the context of citizenship as they inhabit a challenging and liminal positioning between childhood, youth and adulthood and are commonly regarded as citizens-in-the-making. Second, the exploration of such issues was particularly pertinent in light of the introduction of compulsory citizenship education at Key Stages 3 and 4. To some degree this curriculum development reinforced the notion of young teenagers as citizens of the future. Alongside such policy developments there have been a number of contradictory messages from politicians and policy-makers regarding appropriate and acceptable forms of 'active citizenship' for young people to engage in. Policy discourses on active citizenship are bounded by acceptable behaviours and shrouded in restrictive overtones of 'helpful involvement'. Finally, the research sought to focus on young teenagers' perspectives in order to question and challenge the increasing criminalization of the young in dominant policy and media discourses.

Using a teenage-centred mixed-method approach the study focused holistically on teenagers' lived experiences as citizens both inside and out of school. In line with the ethos of the NSSC, participants' perspectives were placed centre stage and their views and experiences were explored in relation to participation in decision-making at school (chapter 4); participation in creative and innovative acts of citizenship outside school (chapter 5); and their inclusion within and exclusion from decision-making in local governance (chapter 6). A spatial analysis was also central to the study as a means of highlighting the ways in which teenagers' engagement (re)shapes places within their school and community. Moreover, the power relations inherent within each of those spaces illustrate the challenges teenagers face in becoming recognized as active citizens. Two key arguments have been put forward concerning teenagers' challenging relationship with citizenship, as well as demonstrating the (often unconventional) ways many teenagers are involved as active citizens. I have argued for a more fluid notion of citizenship where children, young teenagers and adults alike are all viewed as full citizens who engage in different forms of citizenship in a variety of spheres. I also argue for a more cosmopolitan approach to teenagers' citizenship, particularly in relation to the current structure of the citizenship curriculum.

Alternative perspectives on teenagers' citizenship

The following section summarizes three key areas of concern to researchers, policy-makers and practitioners: teenagers as citizens-in-the-present, and their active and creative acts of citizenship both within school and in the wider community.

Teenagers as citizens-in-the-present

What it means to be, act and think like a citizen is problematic. Participants in this study demonstrated a wide variety of ways in which they acted and thought as active citizens both within school and in the wider community. The construction of young teenagers as 'between' childhood, youth and adulthood, however, renders their status as citizens problematic within the context of more conventional spheres of citizenship. As many of the preceding chapters have highlighted, children and young teenagers are commonly regarded as incompetent and incomplete and therefore unable to participate as full and active citizens. In many ways, children and young teenagers are still considered in Kantian terms as passive citizens, not able to engage in forms of active citizenship such as voting. Kant did not intend passive to refer to a lesser status but used the term to suggest that such citizenship was a temporary status (Schapiro, 1999). The connotations associated with being passive do not, however, favour the acts of citizenship in which many teenagers are actively engaged. This notion of passive citizenship problematically remains upheld in the idea that citizenship is tied to participation in the labour market. Consumerism is often viewed as one way in which children and teenagers are afforded citizen status. Through increased spending power and strategic marketing campaigns, teenagers have become valuable contributors to the consumer economy. Nevertheless, defining citizenship in terms of consumerism neglects the exclusion, surveillance and control that many face in shops, malls, villages and town centres. As Aitken (2001) suggests, middle-class consumption patterns have reconstructed the street, denying free public access with spaces being controlled and monitored. This field of study would benefit from greater critical analysis of teenagers' citizenship status as consumers.

Despite the positive contributions that the UNCRC has made in raising the global awareness of both children and teenagers' rights and diverse needs, many teenagers in this study also felt alienated by the construction of teenagers as troublemakers. Indeed, many believed they were denied rights because of the age-based stereotypes in society. Furthermore, others were unaware of the rights that they do have. Evidence presented in this book suggests that many teenagers *do* engage in numerous acts of citizenship at the local or even micro-level, either through the carving out of spaces to hang out in both at school and in the local area, where facilities are not available, or through the regeneration of local areas. At the global level the anti-war demonstrations organized and mobilized by children and teenagers challenge the notion of apathy and demonstrate alternative strategies of resistance and campaign. Indeed, these actions both challenge and quash the notion of teenage apathy and highlight the need for a broader societal acceptance of teenagers as active citizens. As Beck (1992) suggests, societal changes coupled with the decline in affiliation to the nation-state have resulted in new social movements. Such acts of citizenship, both at the local and state level, not only contest adult constructions of childhood but challenge dominant norms of appropriate citizenship for the young. Promoting such practices is challenging in a societal system that represents teenagers as apathetic because they do not necessarily conform to conventional understandings of politics and citizenship. Rather, current policy drives place the focus of disaffection at the level of the individual, hoping that initiatives such as citizenship education will (re)motivate particular young people. Whilst many participants were cynical, this was targeted more at formal political institutions, decision-makers and politicians rather than 'politics' per se (see also Hine *et al.*, 2004). Perhaps this says more about the state of democracy and political institutions than about teenagers' apathy. Meaningful self-reflection on the part of politicians and policy-makers is necessary and requires a move beyond, for example, dressing informally on school visits, to consider a more radical re-conceptualization of teenagers' role in formal politics. Arguably, apathy, as it is commonly defined, is rife across generations.

Young teenagers are not merely excluded by virtue of their age but also by the dominant understandings of citizenship drawn upon and utilized in contemporary British policy, for example, the development of citizenship education. This book has argued for a more flexible and inclusive approach to citizenship, questioning dominant liberal and communitarian understandings for their rigid definition of key elements of citizenship, in particular the focus on citizenship at the level of the nation-state. As France (1998) argues, participating as citizens usually refers to involvement either in liberal democratic institutions and mechanisms or in the community. The adult-centric nature of liberal democracy excludes children and young teenagers from direct representation. Moreover, individualization, Thomas and Hocking (2003) suggest, has further excluded children from mainstream political life. Children and teenagers have no direct link to mainstream politics except through their parents. Cosmopolitan democracy, however, moves away from the idea that citizenship relations are principally state-based, instead focusing upon the local–global nexus (Habermas, 1996; Held, 1996; Held and McGrew, 2000). There are many advantages to taking a more cosmopolitan approach to citizenship, which recognizes the globalized world as dynamic, encapsulating many diverse identities whilst also focusing on the manifestations of these issues at the local level. Nevertheless, propositions for a cosmopolitan citizenship education (see Osler and Starkey, 2003) are centred around notions of respect and peace, and fail to recognize differing and opposing ideas of 'the good' or indeed that active citizenship can be seen as 'oppositional and disruptive' (Lister, 1997b: 33). Isin and Wood's (1999) notion of the 'radical democratic citizen' is perhaps more pertinent to the experiences of many teenagers.

Active and creative citizenship in school

The introduction of compulsory citizenship education in English secondary schools in 2002 has received a mixed response from practitioners and young participants. Whilst citizenship education has raised teenagers' awareness of many issues, a significant proportion of respondents were not engaged in the subject. Nationally, coverage appears to remain patchy, and teachers and schools still need more training and support. The ongoing longitudinal study conducted by the National Foundation for Educational Research will be invaluable in tracking the progress of the subject. Nevertheless, I believe a number of fundamental challenges remain with regard to both the conceptualization of young teenagers' role and status as citizens, as well as the understanding of citizenship underlying the curriculum development. Citizenship education, the 'unfinished political project', remains, to a large degree, incomplete for it fails to tap into teenagers' own experiences. Teenagers' participation and education rights are often ignored within school, where they are treated as morally inferior (Mayall, 2000; 2002). Furthermore, citizenship education's focus on creating *future responsible citizens* reflects broader societal discourses which regard the young as citizens-in-the-making. As Wyness argues:

> The education system still seems to work on the basis that children are both ontologically absent and socially incompetent and therefore unfit to reflect on school choice and policy.
>
> (1999: 366)

This book endorses Osler and Starkey's (2003) criticism that a curriculum built upon the idea of citizens-in-the-making is likely to create further resentment. As Mayall (2002) also observes, those in compulsory schooling are constructed as learners not workers. Citizenship education, therefore, reinforces a non-citizen status. I call for a cumulative notion of citizenship where children, teenagers and adults alike are meaningfully regarded as full citizens who, throughout their life, learn, develop and engage in different forms of citizenship. This study has highlighted the positive outcomes that raising teenagers' status can have upon their engagement with citizenship. When deficit models of childhood and citizenship are disregarded in the classroom, this has a positive effect on engagement with the subject. For example, when teenagers feel that they are treated like adults or perhaps as equals, and where they are afforded the opportunity actively to make decisions over their learning, they are more likely to be engaged in citizenship education. Positive examples of this practice were witnessed, although it must be stated that this is often due to the practices of individual teachers rather than a whole school or nationwide education culture. Alderson (2000b) suggests that children and young people become democratic citizens through practice. Poor examples of citizenship in practice within schools have the potential to disengage teenagers. This has important implications for the way in which education policy constructs future curricula. Nevertheless, the response of some teenagers to educational policy on citizenship is also influenced by other macro systems. For example, on deciding the merit of studying citizenship, concerns were raised over its potential imposition on other curriculum subjects and achievement within exams. This illustrates the broader political and educational contexts in which teenagers' lived experiences are informed and constrained.

Children and teenagers on the anti-war demonstrations were threatened with truancy records for the day (Birkett, 2003). This ultimately throws into question the rationale behind, and the future efficacy of, the government's policy on citizenship education. It is fruitful to draw upon Blaug's (2002) notions of 'incumbent' and 'critical' democracy whereby 'incumbent' democracy refers to compliance, whilst 'critical' democracy refers to alternative forms of citizenship which encompass struggles and protest and may be in opposition to the government (Faulks, 2006). The citizenship curriculum appears to endorse a more incumbent notion of democracy whilst the actions of many teenagers reflect a more critical understanding of democracy. In these terms acts of citizenship which fall outside of more conventional understandings are seldom recognized as worthwhile political engagements. Indeed, rather than the rhetoric of 'active citizenship' (see QCA, 2000), it would appear that both the state and society would prefer only 'helpful involvement' from children and teenagers. The government's quest to reduce teenage apathy is also cautious of the opposing outcomes. To critique the rationale of citizenship education would be to suggest that it is not only about creating future responsible citizens but is also about institutionalizing, controlling and moulding the kind of citizenship in which teenagers may legitimately become engaged, and is certainly not synonymous with Brown's (1997) radical notions of agonistic and antagonistic citizenship. In these more critical terms, citizenship education may be seen as an extension of the state panoptican.

I believe that creating curricula that value and respect teenagers' needs and aspirations, in addition to developing opportunities for teenagers actively to engage with local decision-makers over the issues that are of importance at present, are important steps towards societal respect for teenagers' current personhood, thus inciting confidence that their political actions matter. It is important also to view teenagers as experts in their own citizenship. The curriculum would benefit greatly from taking a more flexible stance to citizenship and from drawing upon teenagers' own engagements with citizenship in order to inform and incite debate and discussion within the classroom (Weller, 2003).

Active and creative citizenship in the wider community

In discussing teenagers' citizenship both in school and in the wider community it is useful to look to Sharp *et al.*'s (2000) notions of dominating and resisting power. They suggest that 'dominating power' refers to control or coercion, whilst 'resisting power' is concerned with the repulsion of dominant forces. These power relations are not simply two-way exchanges but instead may be regarded as a complex network (Foucault, 1977; 1979; 1980; Sharp *et al.*, 2000). It is apparent that many teenagers are controlled not only by the complex stereotypes afforded to them but by the regulation and surveillance that they face within their communities and institutions such as schools (see also James *et al.*, 1998). Many teenagers demonstrated resisting power, creating spaces out of an absence of place, exerting citizenship where they were not afforded it, through clothing, music and lifestyle choices, and creating spaces of citizenship and belonging via sometimes self-directed regeneration projects. This kind of resisting power is a struggle. Teenagers struggle against an adult-dominated society and against resentment and disillusion fostered through a lack of belonging. At the same time, different groups dominate different situations and spaces either within school or within the community. Some may control areas where adults fear to tread. Moreover, local decision-makers may also resist the power that teenagers try to exert. These are not simple power exchanges (see Foucault, 1977; 1979; 1980; Sharp *et al.*, 2000) but may be seen as a complex web of interactions.

The research has highlighted the myriad ways in which teenagers exert their own practises of citizenship in their communities. The stories I have presented detail the lives of a number of teenagers living in a relatively deprived area with limited local facilities and resources. Through their own creativity, innovation and social networks they have succeeded in changing and improving their local environments, thus challenging the notion of teenage apathy. They have established themselves as committed political actors. Many examples of this political action centred on creating spaces for teenagers. Through campaigning for skate-park facilities, revitalizing new spaces to hang out in and maintaining old facilities, many participants demonstrated a more radical or post-modern approach to citizenship. At the national and global level, the anti-war protests organized by children and teenagers in 2003 also highlight significant examples of active citizenship, although these actions are often at odds with the kind of citizenship prescribed in the curriculum. Furthermore, these actions challenge the notion of teenage apathy and highlight the need for a broader societal acceptance of teenagers as active citizens. As Watts argues:

> political interest and participation are not necessarily being abandoned by contemporary youth: they are being redefined, particularly when they conjoin with localised, single-issue and social interests.
>
> (2006: 89)

Many participants also asserted themselves as political actors by drawing attention to new citizen identities based upon lifestyle choices and interests. Many aspects of teenagers' identity were related to different cultural and interest groups. These groups reflected local reconstructions of global youth identities. For example, identities centred on 'townie' youth cultures are common in other areas of England (Haydon, 2002), whilst groups such as skateboarders exert global identities. Such group identities may be referred to in different terms and may occupy different spaces in other locales, but in essence they have global connections through music, clothing (see Swain, 2002) and shared experiences, many of which are connected along global lines of communication. Within school settings, Valentine (2003) suggests, young people must exert individuality whilst at the same time conforming to peer culture. This research has highlighted the complexities in this statement by revealing the multilayered nature of peer group cultures. Moreover, these cultural, lifestyle and interest groups have blurred membership boundaries. Individuals or collectives may buy into more than one group, but often with implications for how they are viewed, included or excluded by others. This demonstrates an individualized consumerism, where an individual can buy into different lifestyle choices. Beck's (1992) writings on individualization help to account for the greater identity and culture choices faced by teenagers. Adopting such identities, he suggests, is risky as it can lead to marginalization. This research certainly highlights that particular groups of teenagers, especially those identifying with skateboard cultures, are especially marginalized by their spatial and lifestyle choices. At the same time, some teenagers choose not to be labelled by one lifestyle or interest, and instead belong to a variety of communities, negotiating different identities at different times. The complex constructions of identity revealed in this study have significant implications for the delineation of teenagers along traditional boundaries for researchers and policy-makers. Whilst categories such as gender, ethnicity and class remain important, an understanding of this alternative context of identity has been essential to exploring teenagers' spaces of citizenship, for they frequently determine their engagement. This study was not able to examine the potential implications of ethnicity in the creation of such identity groups. An examination of urban group identities and citizenship education may prove worthwhile. Nevertheless, local and national government needs to acknowledge the interests, needs and aspirations of teenagers as fractured along traditional lines as well as dispersing amongst new identities. Policy-makers, therefore, need to recognize alternative citizen identities and acts of engagement as valid in order to deter further marginalization.

The majority of teenage participants in this research felt excluded from a variety of social and political spheres within their communities. The overwhelming majority felt excluded from local governance by virtue of their age and subsequent positioning in society. Few teenagers identified a sense of belonging in relation to the conventional construction of community.

Many felt teenagers were often stereotyped as troublemakers. Several believed that local decision-makers neglected the needs of *young* teenagers by not providing suitable and accessible facilities. Moreover, few had been afforded opportunities to participate in local decision-making, and where avenues had been provided the methods of consultation used were limited and rarely meaningful. There was, however, a feeling of resentment between many teenagers and local decision-makers. Despite the lack of participatory opportunities available to teenagers, many participants wanted to be involved in the political mainstream. Local decision-makers play an important role in shaping teenagers' lives, and whilst some, to some extent, have responded to calls for children and teenagers to be consulted, within this local context opportunities for participation were sparse. Where they were available, inappropriate methods of consultation were often adopted and participants seldom received feedback. Many teenagers perceived these consultations to be meaningless and unlikely to result in any real action. This study is limited in its examination of participatory opportunities for young teenagers nationally. Nevertheless, at the level of this case study it is clear that the adoption of the principles of the UNCRC or indeed the philosophies of the NSSC would be beneficial to decision-makers' understandings of teenagers' diverse needs and interests.

In summary, many participants described frustrating spaces of exclusion, of non-belonging, of not being heard, of superficial consultation, of little status and of stereotypes. I would hope there are more inclusive and effective participatory practices in other areas, but this is doubtful within the broader context of local government participation strategies. The guidelines in the government's Green Paper *Every Child Matters* may go some way to aid the development of more meaningful participatory practices (DfES, 2003). Moreover, Thomas and Hocking (2003) argue for the electoral franchise to be extended to those aged 14–17. I suggest that as local areas are of fundamental importance to many teenagers, a practical starting point might be to provide the opportunity for participation in local elections. This is not to suggest that this is the only form of action that should be taken or that all young teenagers would wish to participate in this way. Instead I believe it would not only attempt to increase teenagers' perceived and actual status, but would also help to counter the growing resentment towards local decision-makers at the lack of opportunity for meaningful participation. This must be coupled with recognition of other forms of participation which involve the widespread acknowledgement of different understandings of politics (see O'Toole, 2003) and citizenship. What remains apparent is a fundamental contradiction. Whilst policy-makers are fearful of teenage apathy, they are also fearful of teenagers' political engagement. These are not merely issues for the policies of British government but have broader implications internationally.

Concluding thoughts

As chapter 1 alluded, the 'social' and arguably the 'political' are spatially constructed (Massey *et al.*, 1999). It is, however, relatively uncommon for studies on citizenship to adopt a geographical perspective which investigates citizenship across a number of spatial scales. Competing understandings of citizenship are inherently couched in arguments over space and are tied to questions concerning 'who belongs?' and 'where do they belong?' Such contestations relate to the most appropriate spatial unit of citizenship whether that be the nation-state or a more local or global forum. Developing Foster's (1997) and Lister's (1997a; 1997b) focus on the inclusionary and exclusionary dimensions of dominant understandings of citizenship, it is vital to recognize the spatial manifestations of such inclusion and exclusion in different political institutions. Studies on citizenship also have much to learn from the work of children's geographies and other research *with* children as this approach commonly places emphasis on children as social actors competent in effecting change and shaping their own life-worlds and the environments of others. Drawing upon this conceptual stance has the potential to afford teenagers' status greater parity with that of adults. A geographical gaze, therefore, is fruitful in a number of important dimensions.

A geographical stance reveals much about teenagers' lived relationship with citizenship, highlighting understandings at the global, national and local levels. Space matters at the micro-level as it illuminates teenagers' performative role as citizens. In the main, it is local or micro-spaces that constitute the arenas that motivate, interest, enrage and excite teenagers (Weller, 2003). Such spaces of citizenship are often contested, controversial and unrecognized as legitimate or conventional forms of political engagement and indeed have to be read with a more enlightened understanding of citizenship. Many participants also revealed more global perspectives on citizenship through their identification with, for example, cyberspace and international consumer brands. This again highlights a more cosmopolitan notion of citizenship. It is also likely that if the study had also been conducted in a more urban, cosmopolitan area then participants may have identified other diasporic and multiple understandings of citizenship and identity. It is, however, at the mezzo- or national level that participants felt most disenfranchised from citizenship. It is at this level, the echelon with which politicians and policy-makers are most concerned, that a large proportion of teenagers are most sceptical, particularly because they remain excluded from many mainstream political institutions by virtue of their age. A spatial analysis reveals much about teenagers' alternative, and often hidden, understandings and acts of citizenship. This book, therefore, calls for more emphasis on an explicitly spatial analysis of citizenship that seeks to understand the arenas in which struggles, challenges and conflicts and more radical forms of citizenship occur.

To meaningfully view teenagers as active and equal citizens requires a fundamental shift in societal discourse, which moves beyond the recognition that teenagers are a diverse and competent social group. Such positioning, whilst wholly worthy in promoting teenagers' neglected voices, is now perhaps at risk of reinforcing the adult/child dialectic by segregating their voices and experiences from the 'adult world' (Weller, 2003). This is not to neglect that, as a social group(s), teenagers hold some unique characteristics. At the same time, however, citizenship must move beyond legal and economic terminology, to integrate teenagers as far as possible into the political mainstream, where the diverse thoughts, voices, experiences and competencies of society as a totality are recognized (Weller, 2003). Such a move needs to be coupled with a multi-agency appreciation of the importance of teenagers' lives in the here-and-now rather than as citizens of the future.

Notes

1 The author's doctoral research – 'Teenage Citizenship Geographies: Rural Spaces of Exclusion, Education and Creativity' (Weller, 2004a).
2 Throughout this book the 'modern conceptualization of childhood' refers to the dominant Western conceptualization.
3 As a rural area the minority ethnic population is very low.
4 'Island High' is a pseudonym. To protect the identity of the school, references to the OFSTED report have been omitted.
5 Years 9, 10 and 11 refer to the last three years of compulsory schooling. Participants were, therefore, aged 13–16.
6 GCSE – 'General Certificate of Secondary Education'. Students generally study for GCSEs during years 10–11.
7 The USA and Somalia have expressed an intention to ratify (Osler and Starkey, 2005b).
8 The socially and politically concerned middle-classes.
9 The area operates a three-school system encompassing primary, middle and high schools. Participants, therefore, had experience of a number of schools.
10 *Big Brother* is a television game show where contestants are placed in a house and monitored by cameras for around twelve weeks. Each week the general public votes for one housemate to be evicted. The final housemate wins a cash prize.
11 Reports detailing some of the key findings presented in this book were sent to local decision-makers, the school and participants.
12 Agenda 21 is a global agreement aimed at countering environmental, social and economic problems.

References

Aitken, S.C. (2001) *Geographies of Young People: The Morally Contested Spaces of Identity*, London: Routledge.

Alanen, L. (1994) Gender and generation: feminism and the 'child' question, in Qvortrup, J., Bardy, M., Sgritta, G. and Wintersberger, H. (eds) *Childhood Matters: Social Theory, Practice and Politics*, Aldershot: Avebury Press.

Alanen, L. (1997) Children's childhoods in kinder und kindheit, *Childhood*, Vol. 4(2), pp.251–256.

Alderson, P. (1995) *Listening to Children: Children, Ethics and Social Research*, Barkingside: Barnados.

Alderson, P. (2000a) Children as researchers: the effects of participation rights on research methodology, in Christensen, P. and James, A. (eds) *Research with Children: Perspectives and Practices*, London: Falmer Press, pp.241–257.

Alderson, P. (2000b) School students' views on school councils and daily life, *Children & Society*, Vol. 14, pp.121–134.

Alderson, P. (2000c) *Young Children's Rights: Exploring Beliefs, Principles and Practice*, London: Jessica Kingsley.

Alderson, P. (2002) Students' rights in British schools: trust, autonomy, connection and regulation, in Edwards, R. (ed.) *Children, Home and School: Regulation, Autonomy or Connection?* London: Routledge, pp.24–40.

Alexander, G. (1995) Children's rights in their early years: from plaiting fog to knitting treacle, in Franklin, B. (ed.) *The Handbook of Children's Rights: Comparative Policy and Practice*, London: Routledge, Chapter 10.

Allen, J. with the collective (1999) Afterword: open geographies, in Massey, D., Allen, J. and Sarre, P. (eds) *Human Geography Today*, Cambridge: Polity, pp.323–328.

Archard, D. (1993) *Children: Rights and Childhood*, London: Routledge.

Aries, P. (1962) *Centuries of Childhood*, New York: Vintage Press.

Armstrong–Esther, D. and Goodwin, M. (2003) *Meeting the health needs of rural young people through evaluating their experience of community*, Youthful Ruralities Seminar, University of Swansea, 19th February.

Attwood, C., Singh, G., Prime, D. and Creasey, R. (2003) *2001 Home Office Citizenship Survey: People, Families and Communities*, Home Office Research Study 270, London: Home Office.

Audi, R. (1996) *The Cambridge Dictionary of Philosophy*, Cambridge: CUP.

Baggini, J. (2002) *Philosophy: Key Themes*, Basingstoke: Palgrave Macmillan.

Baginsky, M. and Hannam, D. (1999) *School Councils: The Views of Students and Teachers*, http://www.nspcc.org.uk/Inform/Research/Findings/SchoolCouncils_asp_ifega26204.html, accessed 11th December 2006.

Barker, J. and Weller, S. (2003a) 'Never work with children?': The geography of methodological issues in research with children, *Qualitative Research*, Vol. 3(2), pp.207–227.

Barker, J. and Weller, S. (2003b) 'Is it fun?' Developing children centred research methods, *International Journal of Sociology and Social Policy*, Vol. 23 (1/2), pp.33–59.

Barnett, C. and Low, M. (2004) Geography and democracy: an introduction, Barnett, C. and Low, M. (eds) *Spaces of Democracy: Geographical Perspectives on Citizenship, Participation and Representation*, London: Sage, pp.1–22.

Barton, L. (2002) A room of their own, *Guardian Education*, 29th October, p.7.

BBC (2003a) *Hodge is Minister for Children*, http://news.bbc.co.uk/1/hi/education/2988734.stm, accessed 3rd April 2004.

BBC (2003b) *Mother loses contraceptive test case*, http://news.bbc.co.uk/onthisday/low/dates/stories/july/26/newsid_2499000/2499583.stm, accessed 11th November 2003.

BBC (2006) *Guide to comedy: the Catherine Tate show*, http://www.bbc.co.uk/comedy/guide/articles/c/catherinetateshow_999040216.shtml, accessed 21st June 2006.

Beck, U. (1992) *Risk Society: Towards a New Modernity*, London: Sage.

Beck, U. (2000) *What is Globalization?* Translated by Patrick Camiller, Cambridge: Polity Press.

Bedell, G. (2003) *Voices of tomorrow don't wait to protest*, http://www.observer.co.uk/children/story/0,12816,920067,00.html, accessed 5th May 2003.

Beetham, D. and Boyle, K. (1998) What is Democracy? in Giddens, A. (ed.) *Sociology: Introductory Readings*, Cambridge: Polity.

Bennett, A. (1999) Subcultures of neo-tribes? Rethinking the relationship between youth, style and musical taste, *Sociology*, Vol. 33(3), pp.599–617.

Bhattacharyya, G. (2004) Practical citizenship, *Guardian Unlimited*, 10th June, http://education.guardian.co.uk/print/0,3858,4944017–110979,00.html, accessed 8th February 2005.

Biesta, G. and Lawy, R. (2006) From teaching citizenship to learning democracy: overcoming individualism in research, policy and practice, *Cambridge Journal of Education*, Vol. 36(1), pp.63–79.

Bingham, N., Valentine, G. and Holloway, S.L. (1999) Where do you want to go tomorrow? Connecting children and the internet, *Environment and Planning D: Society and Space*, Vol. 17, pp.655–672.

Birkett, D. (2003) It's their war too, *Guardian Education*, 25th March, pp.2–3.

Blaug, R. (2002) Engineering democracy, *Political Studies*, Vol. 50(1), pp.102–116.

Blaut, J. and Stea, D. (1971) Studies of geographic learning, *Annals of the Association of American Geographers*, Vol. 61, pp.387–449.

Borden, I. (2001) *Skateboarding, Space and the City: Architecture and the Body*, Oxford: BERG.

Brighouse, H. (1998) Civic education and liberal legitimacy, *Ethics*, Vol. 108(4), pp.719–746.

Bright, M. and Dodd, V. (1998) Pupils face 'good citizen' class, *The Observer*, 15th March, p.19.

Brown, M.P. (1997) *Replacing Citizenship: Aids, Activism and Radical Democracy*, London: The Guildford Press.

Bunge, W. (1973) The point of reproduction: a second front, *Antipode*, Vol. 9, pp.60–76.

Bunting, M. (2004) Teen troubles: questions still unanswered, *The Guardian*, 13th September, p.4.

Burrell, I. (2001) Curfew law impossible to enforce, say campaigners, *The Independent*, 2nd August, p.8.

Cahill, C. (2000) Street literacy: urban teenagers' strategies for negotiating their neighbourhood, *Journal of Youth Studies*, Vol. 3(3), pp.251–277.

Chawla, L. (2001) Putting young old ideas into action: the relevance of growing up in cities to Local Agenda 21, *Local Environment*, Vol. 6(1), pp.13–25.

Chisholm, L. (2001) Critical discussion: from the margins – the darker side of empowerment, in Helve, H. and Wallace, C. (eds) *Youth, Citizenship and Empowerment*, Aldershot: Ashgate, pp.129–138.

Chrisafis, A. (2002) Get with it, *The Guardian G2 Supplement*, 18th January, pp.2–3.

Christensen, P. James, A. and Jenks, C. (2000) *Changing Times: Children's Understandings of the Social Organisation of Time*, Children 5–16 Research Briefing, No. 15, Swindon: ESRC.

Citizenship Foundation (2000) *Citizenship and the National Curriculum*, http://www.citizenshipfoundation.org.uk/main/page.php?6, accessed 2nd February 2001.

Cleaver, E., Ireland, E., Kerr, D. and Lopes, J. (2005) Listening to young people: citizenship education in England, *Citizenship Education Longitudinal Study: Second Cross-Sectional Survey 2004 – Research Brief: RB626*, Nottingham: DfES.

Clemitshaw, G. and Calvert, M. (2005) Implementing citizenship in the English secondary school curriculum: a follow-up study, *Pastoral Care*, Vol. 23(3), pp.31–36.

Cockburn, T. (1998) Children and citizenship in Britain: a case for a socially independent model of citizenship, *Childhood*, 5(1) pp.99–117.

Cockburn, T. (2000) From 'street Arabs' to 'angels': working-class children, competence and citizenship, 1850–1914, in Batsleer, J. and Humphries, B. (eds) *Welfare, Exclusion and Political Agency*, London: Routledge, pp.22–46.

Cogan, J.J. (2000) Citizenship education for the 21st century: setting the context, in Cogan, J.J. and Derricott, R. (eds) *Citizenship for the 21st Century: An International Perspective on Education*, London: Kogan Page, pp.1–22.

Commission on Citizenship (1990) *Encouraging Citizenship*, London: HMSO.

Connexions (2004) *At what age can I?* http://www.connexions-direct.com/index.cfm?pid=161andcatalogueContentID=176andrender=detailedArticle, accessed 21st December 2004.

Corsaro, W.A. (1997) *The Sociology of Childhood*, Thousand Oaks, CA: Pine Forge Press.

Countryside Agency (2000) *The State of the Countryside 2000*, Cheltenham: Countryside Agency.

Countryside Agency (2003a) *The State of the Countryside 2003*, Wetherby, West Yorkshire: Countryside Agency.

Countryside Agency (2003b) *The Implementation of Connexions in Rural Areas*, Cheltenham: Countryside Agency.

Crace, J. (2000) The new citizens, *Guardian Education*, 15th February , pp.2–3.

Crace, J. (2004) Absolutely positive, *The Guardian*, 7th September, http://education.guardian.co.uk/egweekly/story/0,,1298259,00.html, accessed 7th September 2004.

Crace, J. (2005) Life's what you make it, *The Guardian*, 25th January, http://education.guardian.co.uk/print/0,3858,5110565–110908,00.html, accessed 24th February 2005.

Crick, B. (2000) *Essays on Citizenship*, London: Continuum.

Crick, B. (2002) Education for citizenship: the Citizenship Order, *Parliamentary Affairs*, Vol. 55(3), pp.488–504.

Crow, M. (2004) Citizenship classes 'need more support', *Guardian Unlimited*, 7th September, http://education.guardian.co.uk/print/0,3858,5010138-110908,00.html, accessed 24th February 2005.

Cunningham, S. and Lavalette, M. (2004) 'Active citizens' or 'irresponsible truants'? School student strikes against the war, *Critical Social Policy*, Vol. 24(2), pp.255–269.

CYPU (2001) *Learning to Listen: Core Principles for the Involvement of Children and Young People*, Annesley, Nottinghamshire: DfES.

CYPU (2002) *Young People and Politics*, London: CYPU.

Davies, B. and Marken, M. (2000) All those in favour ..., *Young People Now*, April, pp.30–32.

Davies, I., Gregory, I. and Shirley, R.C. (1999) *Good Citizenship and Education Provision*, London: Falmer Press.

Davis, M. (1990) *City of Quartz*, London: Verso.

Delfos, M. (2001) *Are You Listening to Me? Communicating with Children from Four to Twelve Years*, Amsterdam: SWP, Amsterdam.

DETR (1998) *Modern Local Government: In Touch with the People*, White Paper, CM4014, London: HMSO.

De Waal, A. (2002) 'Realising child rights in Africa: children, young people and leadership', in De Waal, A. and Argenti, N. (eds) *Young Africa: Realising the Rights of Children and Youth*, Trenton, NJ: Africa World Press, pp.1–28.

Dewey, J. (1916) *Democracy and Education*, 1966 edition, New York: Free Press.

DfEE (1997) *Excellence in Schools*, White Paper, London: Stationery Office.

DfEE (2000) *Citizenship for 16–19 year olds in Education and Training*, Coventry: Further Education Funding Council.

DfEE and QCA (1999) *Citizenship: The National Curriculum for England – Key Stages 3–4*, London: DfEE and QCA.

DfES (2003) *Every Child Matters*, www.everychildmatters.gov.uk, accessed 1st April 2004.

DfES (2006) *Citizenship: The National Curriculum for England*, http://www.dfes.gov.uk/citizenship/, accessed 14th August 2006.

Dillabough, J-A. and Arnot, M. (2000) (eds) *Challenging Democracy: International Perspectives on Gender, Education and Citizenship*, London: Routledge.

DTI (2005) *The National Minimum Wage*, http://www.dti.gov.uk/employment/pay/national-minimum-wage/index.html, accessed 11th December 2006.

Duffy, M. (1996) Schools can't compensate for society, *New Statesman*, Vol. 129 (4517), p.23.

Dwyer, P. (2004) *Understanding Social Citizenship: Themes and Perspectives for Policy and Practice*, Bristol: Policy Press.

Edwards, R. (2002) (ed.) *Children, Home and School: Regulation, Autonomy or Connection?* London: Routledge.

Edwards, J. and Fogelman, K. (1991) Active citizenship and young people, in Fogelman, K. (ed) *Citizenship in Schools*, London: David Fulton, pp.17–34.

Enfield, H. (1997) *Harry Enfield and his Humorous Chums*, London: Penguin.

Ennew, J. (1994) Time for children or time for adults? in Qvortrup, J., Bardy, M., Sgritta, G. and Wintersberger, H. (eds) *Childhood Matters: Social Theory, Practice and Politics*, Aldershot: Avebury, pp.125–143.

ESRC (2005) *Low election turnout reflects the failure of UK politicians*, http://www.esrcsocietytoday.ac.uk/ESRCInfoCentre/PO/releases/2005/June/index5.aspx, accessed 21st June 2006.

Euronet (2000) *Euronet Report*, http://www.europeanchildrensnetwork.org/Documents/EuronetRep1.htm, accessed 1st November 2000.

Faulks, K. (1998) *Citizenship in Modern Citizenship*, Edinburgh: Edinburgh University Press.

Faulks, K. (2000) *Citizenship*, London: Routledge.

Faulks, K. (2006) Education for citizenship in England's secondary schools: a critique of current principle and practice, *Journal of Education Policy*, Vol. 21(1), pp.59–74.

Flew, A. (2000) *Education for Citizenship*, London: IEA.

Foley, P. and Martin, S. (2000) A new deal for the community? Public participation in regeneration and local service delivery, *Policy and Politics*, Vol. 28(4), pp.479–491.

Foster, V. (1997) Feminist theory and the construction of citizenship education, in Kennedy, K.J. (ed.) *Citizenship Education and the Modern State*, London: Falmer Press, pp.54–64.

Foucault, M. (1977) *Discipline and Punishment*, London: Allen Lane.

Foucault, M. (1979) *The History of Sexuality Vol.1*, New York: Vintage Books.

Foucault, M. (1980) *Power/Knowledge: Selected Interviews & Other Writings 1972–1977* (Gordon, C. (ed.)), London: Harvester.

France, A. (1998) 'Why should we care?' Young people, citizenship and questions of social responsibility, *Journal of Youth Studies*, Vol. 1(1), pp.97–111.

Fraser, N. (1997) *Justice Interruptus: Critical Reflections on the 'Postsocialist' Condition*, London: Routledge.

Freeman, C. (1999) Children's participation in environmental decision-making, in Buckingham-Hatfield, S. and Percy, S. (eds) *Constructing Local Environmental Agendas: People, Places and Participation*, London: Routledge, pp.68–80.

Freeman, C., Nairn, K., and Sligo, J. (2003) 'Professionalizing' participation from rhetoric to practice, *Children's Geographies*, Vol. 1(1), pp.53–70.

Freie, J.F. (1998) *Counterfeit Community: The Exploration of Our Longings for Connectedness*, Maryland: Rowman and Littlefield.

Gerrard, N. (1999) Innocence on the line, *The Observer*, 14th November, p.1.

Gibbs, D.C., Jonas, A.E.G., Reimer, S. and Spooner, D.J. (2001) Governance, institutional capacity and partnerships in local economic development: theoretical issues and empirical evidence from the Humber sub-region, *Transactions of the Institute of British Geographers*, Vol. 26(1), pp.103–120.

Giddens, A. (2000a) *Runaway World*, New York: Routledge.

Giddens, A. (2000b) Citizenship in a global era, in Pearce, N. and Hallgarten, J. (eds) *Tomorrow's Citizens*, London: IPPR, pp.17–25.

Gifford, C. (2004) National and post-national dimensions of citizenship education in the UK, *Citizenship Studies*, Vol. 8(2), pp.145–158.

Gittens, D. (1998) *The Child in Question*, Basingstoke: Macmillan.

Gordon, T., Holland, J. and Lehelma, E. (2000) *Making Spaces: Citizenship and difference in schools*, Basingstoke: Macmillan.

Gould, C. (1988) *Rethinking Democracy*, Cambridge: CUP.

Greig, A. and Taylor, J. (1999) *Doing Research with Children*, London: Sage.

Griffith, R. (1998) *Educational Citizenship and Independent Learning*, London: Jessica Kingsley.

Grosvenor, I. and Lawn, M. (2004) Days out of school: secondary education, citizenship and public space in 1950s England, *History of Education*, Vol. 33(4), pp.377–389.

Habermas, J. (1996) *Between Facts and Norms*, London: Polity.

Hahn, C.L. (1999) Citizenship education: an empirical study of policy, practices and outcomes, *Oxford Review of Education*, Vol. 25(1&2), pp.231–250.

Halfacree, K. (1996a) Trespassing against the rural idyll: the Criminal Justice and Public Order Act 1994 and access to the countryside, in Watkins, C. (ed.) *Rights of Way*, London: Pinter.

Halfacree, K. (1996b) Out of place in the country: travellers and the rural idyll, *Antipode*, 28, pp.42–72.

Hall, T., Coffey, A. and Williamson, H. (1999) Self, space and place: youth identities and citizenship, *British Journal of Sociology of Education*, Vol. 20(4), pp.501–513.

Halpern, D., John, P. and Morris, Z. (2002) Before the Citizenship Order: a survey of citizenship education practice in England, *Journal of Education Policy*, Vol. 17(2), pp.217–228.

Harkin, J. (2005) Active citizenship, *The Guardian*, 5th November, http://www.guardian.co.uk/print/0,,5326560-103677,00.html, accessed 21st June 2006.

Hart, R. (1984) The geography of children and children's geographies, in Saarinen, T.F., Seamon, D. and Sell, J.L. (eds) *Environmental Perception and Behaviour: An Inventory and Prospect*, University of Chicago, Department of Geography Research Paper No. 209, pp.99–129.

Hart, R. (1992) *Children's Participation: from Tokenism to Participation*, Innocenti Essays, No. 4, Florence: UNICEF.

Hart, R. (1997) *Children's Participation: The Theory and Practice of Involving Young Citizens in Community Development and Environmental Care*, London: UNICEF.

Haydon, C. (2002) D'ya wanna be in my gang? *The Independent*, 31st October, pp.4–5.

Heater, D. (1990) *Citizenship*, London: Longman.

Heater, D. (2001) The history of citizenship education in England, *The Curriculum Journal*, Vol. 12(1), pp.103–123.

Hebdige, D. (1988) *Hiding in the Light: On Images and Things*, London: Routledge.

Held, D. (1995) Democracy and the new international order, in Archibugi, D. and Held, D. (eds) *Cosmopolitan Democracy*, Cambridge: Polity, Chapter 4.

Held, D. (1996) *Models of Democracy*, Cambridge: Polity.

Held, H. and McGrew, A. (2000) *The Global Transformations Reader: An Introduction to the Globalization Debate*, Cambridge: Polity.

Helve, H. and Wallace, C. (2001) (eds) *Youth, Citizenship and Empowerment*, Aldershot: Ashgate.

Hendrick, H. (1997) Constructions and reconstructions of British childhood: an interpretive survey, 1900 to the present, in James, A. and Prout, A. (eds) *Constructing and Reconstructing Childhood*, London: Falmer Press, pp.34–62.

Hey, V. (1997) *The Company She Keeps: An Ethnography of Girls' Friendship*, Buckingham: Open University Press.

Heywood, A. (1992) *Political Ideologies: An Introduction*, Basingstoke: Macmillan.

Hill, F. and Michelson, W. (1981) Towards a geography of urban children and youth, in Herbert, D.T. and Johnston, R.H. (eds) *Geography and the Urban Environment: Progress in Research and Applications*, Vol. 6, Chichester: John Wiley, pp.193–228.

Hine, J., Lemetti, F. and Trikha, S. (2004) Citizenship: young people's perspectives, *Home Office Development and Practice Report 10*, London: Home Office.

Holland, S. (2001) Representing children in child protection assessments, *Childhood*, Vol. 8(3), pp.322–339.

Hollis, R. (1995) *A Geographer's Look at the Isle of Wight*, Newport, Isle of Wight: Cross Publishing.

Holloway, S.L. and Valentine, G. (2000a) (eds) *Children's Geographies: Playing, Living, Learning*, London: Routledge.

Holloway, S.L. and Valentine, G. (2000b) Spatiality and the new social studies of childhood, *Sociology*, Vol. 34(4), pp.763–783.

Holloway, S.L. and Valentine, G. (2003) *Cyberkids: Children in the Information Age*, London: Routledge Falmer.

Holmes, R.M. (1998) *Fieldwork with Children*, London: Sage.

Horelli, L. (1998) Creating child-friendly environments: case studies on children's participation in three European countries, *Childhood*, Vol. 5(2), pp.225–239.

Hudson, A. (2005) Citizenship education and students' identities: a school-based action research project, in Osler, A. (ed.) *Teachers, Human Rights and Diversity*, Stoke on Trent: Trentham, pp.115–132.

Inman, K. (1999) A fair start in life, *The Guardian*, 15th September, pp.6–7.

Ireland, E. and Kerr, D. (2004) Learning from current approaches in schools, *Teaching Citizenship*, Vol. 9, pp.20–25.

Ireland, E., Kerr, D., Lopes, J. and Nelson, J. with Cleaver, E. (2006a) Active citizenship and young people: opportunities, experiences and challenges in and beyond school, *Citizenship Education Longitudinal Study: Fourth Annual Report – DfES Research Report RR732*, Nottingham: DfES.

Ireland, E., Kerr, D., Lopes, J. and Nelson, J. (2006b) Active citizenship and young people: opportunities, experiences and challenges in and beyond school, *Citizenship Education Longitudinal Study: Fourth Annual Report – Research Brief: RB732*, Nottingham: DfES.

Isin, E.F. and Wood, P.K. (1999) *Citizenship and Identity*, London: Sage.

Islandbreaks (2003) www.islandbreaks.co.uk/home/faqs.asp, accessed 31st December 2003.

IWCP (2002a) Helping to drive down crime on the buses, *Isle of Wight County Press*, 22nd November, Spotlight on Youth Section.

IWCP (2002b) Stronger voice for youngsters planned, *Isle of Wight County Press*, 22nd November, Spotlight on Youth Section.

iwight (2002) *Isle of Wight Social Inclusion Strategy 2001–2005*, http://www.iwight.com/council/committees/Mod-Education/10-12-01/Social%20Inclusion%20Strategy%20(version3).htm, accessed 28th January 2002.

James, S. (1990) Is there a 'place' for children in geography? *Area*, 22(3), pp.278–283.

James, A. and James, A.L. (2004) *Constructing Childhood: Theory, Policy and Social Practice*, Basingstoke: Palgrave Macmillan.

James, A., Jenks, C. and Prout, A. (1998) *Theorising Childhood*, Cambridge: Polity.

Jenks, C. (1996) *Childhood*, London: Routledge.

Jenks, C. (2001) The pacing and timing of children's bodies, in Hultqvist, K. and Dahlberg, G. (eds) *Governing the Child in the New Millennium*, London: Routledge Falmer, pp.68–84.

Jochum, V., Pratten, B. and Wilding, K. (2005) *Civil Renewal and Active Citizenship: A Guide to the Debate*, London: NCVO.

Jodry, C. (1997) *Youth Participation and the Role of ANACEJ*, Paper presented at the Congress of Local and Regional Authorities of Europe, Budapest, October.

Johnston, R.J., Gregory, D., Pratt, G. and Watts, M. (2000) *The Dictionary of Human Geography*, Oxford: Blackwell.

Jowell, R. and Park, A. (1998) *Young People, Politics and Citizenship – A Disengaged Generation?* London: The Citizenship Foundation.

JRF (2002) Involving young people in local authority decision-making, *Findings*, York: Joseph Rowntree Foundation.

Keele (2003) *Civil and Family Law*, http://www.keele.ac.uk/depts/so/youthchron/Civil FamilyLaw/8090civfamlaw.htm, accessed 11th November 2003.

Kellet, M. (2005) *How to Develop Children as Researchers: A Step-by-step Guide to Teaching the Research Process*, London: Paul Chapman.

Kennedy, D. (1998) Empathic childrearing and the adult construction of childhood: a psychohistorical look, *Childhood*, Vol. 5(1), pp.9–22.

Kennedy, D. (2000) *Notes on the philosophy of childhood and the politics of subjectivity*, http://www.bu.edu/wcp/Papers/Chil/ChilKenn.htm, accessed 1st November 2000.

Kerr, D. (1999a) Changing the political culture: the advisory group on education for citizenship and the teaching of democracy in schools, *Oxford Review of Education*, Vol. 25 (1&2), pp.275–284.

Kerr, D. (1999b) Citizenship Education: an international comparison, *International Review of Curriculum and Assessment Frameworks*, London: QCA.

Kerr, D., Lines, A., Blenkinsop, S. and Schagen, I. (2002) *England's Results from the IEA International Citizenship Education Study: What Citizenship and Education Mean to 14 Year Olds*, DfES Research Report No. 375, London: Stationery Office.

Kerr, D., Cleaver, E., Ireland, E. and Blenkinsop, S. (2003) *Citizenship Education Longitudinal Study First Cross-Sectional Survey 2001–2002*, Brief No. 416, London: DfES.

Kerr, D., Ireland, E., Lopes, J. and Graig, R. with Cleaver, E. (2004) *Making Citizenship Real: Citizenship Education Longitudinal Study Second Annual Report*, London: DfES.

Khan, S. (2003) Escape to a kid-free village, *The Observer*, 4th May, p.6.

Kingston, P. (2002) Voters in sight, *Guardian Education*, 8th January, p.50.

Kjørholt, A.T. (2004) *Childhood as a Social and Symbolic Space: Discourses on Children as Social Participants in Society*, Doctoral thesis, Trondheim: Norwegian University of Science and Technology, NTNU.

Klaushofer, A. (2002) Vote Early, *Guardian Society*, 28th August, pp.2–3.

Kraack, A. and Kenway, J. (2002) Place, time and stigmatized youthful identities: bad boys in paradise, *Journal of Rural Studies*, 18, pp.145–155.

Krimerman, L. (2001) Participatory action research: should social inquiry be conducted democratically? *Philosophy of the Social Sciences*, Vol. 31(1), pp.60–82.

Laegran, A.S. (2002) The petrol station and the internet cafe: rural technospaces for youth, *Journal of Rural Studies*, 18, pp.157–168.

Lansdown, G. (1994) Children's rights, in Mayall, B. (ed.) *Children's Childhoods Observed and Experienced*, London: Falmer, pp.33–44.

Lansdown, G. (1995) *Taking Part: Children's Participation in Decision-Making*, London: IPPR.

Lawson, H. (2001) Active citizenship in schools and the community, *The Curriculum Journal*, Vol. 12 (2), pp.163–178.

Lawton, D., Cairns, J. and Gardner, R. (2000) *Education for Citizenship*, London: Continuum.

Lefebvre, H. (1991) *The Production of Space*, Oxford: Blackwell.

Leighton, R. (2004) The nature of citizenship education provision: an initial study, *The Curriculum Journal*, Vol. 15(2), pp.167–181.

Leyshon, M. (2002) On being 'in the field': practice, progress and problems in research with young people in rural areas, *Journal of Rural Studies*, 18, pp.179–191.

Lindsay, G. (2000) Researching children's perspectives: ethical issues, in Lewis, A. and Lindsay, G. (eds) *Researching with Children*, Buckingham: Open University Press, pp.1–20.

Lister, R. (1997a) *Citizenship: Feminist Perspectives*, Basingstoke: Macmillan.

Lister, R. (1997b) Citizenship: towards a feminist synthesis, *Feminist Review*, No. 57, Autumn 1997, pp.28–48.

Lister, R. (1998) New conceptions of citizenship, in Ellison, N. and Pierson, C. (eds) *Developments in British Social Policy*, Basingstoke: Macmillan, pp.46–60.

Lister, R., Middleton, S. and Smith, N. (2001) *Young People's Voices: Citizenship Education*, Leicester: NYA.

Lister, R., Smith, N., Middleton, S. and Cox, L. (2003) Young people talk about citizenship: empirical perspectives on theoretical and political debates, *Citizenship Studies*, Vol. 7 (2), pp.235–253.

Literacy Trust (2001) *Sure Start and Sure Start Plus*, http://www.literacytrust. org.uk/Database/early.html, accessed 6th February 2001.

Maffesoli, M. (1996) *The Time of the Tribes: The Decline of Individualism in Mass Society*, London: Sage.

Mahon, A., Clarke, K. and Craig, G. (1996) Researching children: methods and ethics, *Children and Society*, Vol. 10, pp.145–154.

Malik, M. (2002) Pupil power is good for all, *Evening Standard*, 12th February.

Marchant, R. and Kirby, P. (2004) The participation of young children: communication, consultation and involvement, in Neale, B. (ed.) *Young Children's Citizenship*, York: Joseph Rowntree Foundation, pp.92–158.

Marshall, T.H. (1950) *Citizenship and Social Class*, Cambridge: CUP.

Marshall, T.H. (1965) *Social Policy in the Twentieth Century*, London: Hutchinson.

Marston, S.A. and Mitchell, K. (2004) Citizens and the state: citizenship formations in time and space, in Barnett, C. and Low, M. (eds) *Spaces of Democracy: Geographical Perspectives on Citizenship, Participation and Representation*, London: Sage, pp.93–112.

Martindale, A. (1994) The child in the picture: a medieval perspective, in Wood, D. (ed.) *The Church and Childhood, Studies in Church History*, Vol. 31, Oxford: Blackwell, pp.197–232.

Mason, J. (1996) *Qualitative Researching*, London: Sage.

Massey, D. (1993) Power-geometry and a progressive sense of place, in Bird, J., Curtis, B., Putnam, F., Robertson, G. and Tickner, L. (eds) *Mapping the Futures: Local Cultures, Global Change*, London: Routledge, pp.59–69.

Massey, D. with the collective (1999) The 'nature' of human geography: issues and debates, in Massey, D., Allen, J. and Sarre, P. (eds) *Human Geography Today*, Cambridge: Polity, pp.1–21.

Matthews, H. (1992) *Making Sense of Place: Children's Understandings of Large-Scale Environments*, Hemel Hempstead: Harvester Wheatsheaf.

Matthews, H. (2001) Power games and moral territories: ethical dilemmas when working with children and young people, *Ethics, Place, and Environment*, Vol. 4(2), pp.117–178.

Matthews, H. (2003) Coming of age for children's geographies: inaugural editorial, *Children's Geographies*, Vol. 1(1), pp.3–5.

Matthews, H. and Limb, M. (1998) The right to say: the development of youth councils/forums within the UK, *Area*, Vol. 30(1), pp.66–78.

Matthews, H. and Limb, M. (1999) Defining an agenda for the geography of children: review and prospect, *Progress in Human Geography*, Vol. 23(1), pp.61–90.

Matthews, H., Limb, M. and Taylor, M. (1998a) The geography of children: some ethical and methodological considerations for project and dissertation work, *Journal of Geography in Higher Education*, Vol. 22(3), pp.311–324.

Matthews, H. Limb, M. and Percy-Smith, B. (1998b) Changing worlds: the micro-geographies of young teenagers, *Tijdschrift voor Economische en Sociale Geografie*, Vol. 89 (2), pp.193–202.

Matthews, H., Limb, M. and Taylor, M., (1999) Young people's participation and representation in society, *Geoforum*, 30, pp.135–144.

Matthews, H., Taylor, M., Percy-Smith, B. and Limb, M. (2000a) The unacceptable flaneur: the shopping mall as a teenage hangout, *Childhood*, Vol. 7(3), pp.279–294.

Matthews, H., Taylor, M., Sherwood, K., Tucker, F. and Limb, M. (2000b) Growing up in the countryside: children in the rural idyll, *Journal of Rural Studies*, 16, pp.141–153.

Mattingly, D. (2001) Place, teenagers and representations: lessons from a community theatre project, *Social and Cultural Geography*, Vol. 2(4), pp.445–459.

Mauthner, M. (1997) Methodological aspects of collecting data from children: lessons from three research projects, *Children and Society*, Vol. 11, pp.16–28.

Mayall, B. (2000) *Negotiating Childhoods*, Children 5–16 Research Briefing No. 13, Swindon: ESRC.

Mayall, B. (2002) *Towards a Sociology for Childhood*, Buckingham: Open University Press.

McCulloch, K. (2000) Young citizens: youth work, civic participation and the renewal of democracy, *Youth & Policy*, No. 68, pp.34–45.

McGrew, A. (2000) Democracy beyond borders? in Held, D. and McGrew, A. (eds) *The Global Transformations Reader: An Introduction to the Globalization Debate*, Cambridge: Polity, pp.405–419.

Mendick, R. (2002) Child curfews: 'A total failure', *The Independent on Sunday*, 6th January, p.8.

Merrifield, A. (2000) Henri Lefebvre: a socialist in space, in Crang, M. and Thrift, N. (eds) *Thinking Space*, London: Routledge, pp.167–182.

Miles, S. (2000) *Youth Lifestyles in a Changing World*, Buckingham: Open University Press.

Millar, F. (2004) People worth listening to, *The Guardian*, 20th January, http://education.guardian.co.uk/print/0,3858,4839323-111774,00.html, accessed 22nd January 2004.

Miller, P.J. (1982) Psychology and the child, in Rooke, P.T. and Schnell, R.L. (eds) *Studies in Childhood History: A Canadian History*, Calgary: Detselig Enterprises Ltd, pp.57–80.

Miller, J. (1996) *Never Too Young: How Young Children Can Take Responsibility and Make Decisions*, London: Save the Children.

Moggach, T. (2006) Every voice matters, *The Guardian*, 6th June.

Monahan, J. (2002) A bright future for Bradford's youth, *Guardian Education*, 1st October, p.54.

MORI (2001) *Most young people want a greater say in public decision-making*, http://www.ipsos-mori.com/polls/2001/carnegie.shtml, accessed 11th December 2006.

Morrell, F. (1991) The work of the speaker's commission and its definition of citizenship, in Fogelman, K. (ed.) *Citizenship in Schools*, London: David Fulton, pp.6–16.

Morrow, G. and Richards, M. (1996) The ethics of social research with children: an overview, *Children and Society*, 10, pp.90–105.

Morrow, V. (2000) 'Dirty looks' and 'trampy places' in young people's accounts of community and neighbourhood: implications for health inequalities, *Critical Public Health*, Vol. 10(2), pp.141–152.

Morrow, V. (2003) Improving the neighbourhood for children: possibilities and limitations of social capital discourses, in Christensen, P. and O'Brien, M. (eds) *Children in the City: Home, Neighbourhood and Community*, London: Routledge Falmer, pp.162–183.

Mouffe, C. (1992) (ed.) *Dimensions of Democracy*, London: Verso.

Muscroft, S. (1999) (ed.) *Children's Rights: Reality or Rhetoric?: The UN Convention on the Rights of the Child: The First Ten Years*, London: Save the Children Alliance.

Neale, B. (2004) Introduction: young children's citizenship, in Neale, B. (ed.) *Young Children's Citizenship*, York: Joseph Rowntree Foundation, pp.6–18.

Nelson, J. and Kerr, D. (2005) *Active Citizenship: Definitions, Goals and Practices*, http://www.nfer.ac.uk/publications/other-publications/downloadable-reports/active-citizenship-definitions-goals-and-practices.cfm, accessed 3rd August 2006.

Oakley, A. (1994) Women and children first and last: parallels and differences between children's and women's studies, in Mayall, B. (ed.) *Children's Childhoods: Observed and Experienced*, London: Falmer Press, pp.13–32.

O'Brien, M., Jones, D., Sloan, D. and Rustin, M. (2000) Children's independent spatial mobility in the urban public realm, *Childhood*, Vol. 7(3), pp.257–277.

Odone, C. (2002) Idle hands, idle minds, *The Observer*, 6th January, pp.22.

OFSTED (2003) *National Curriculum Citizenship: Planning & Implementation 2002/3*, June 2003, London: OFSTED.

O'Kane, C. (2000) The development of participatory techniques: facilitating children's views about decisions which affect them, in Christensen, P. and James, A. (eds) *Research with Children: Perspectives and Practices*, London: Falmer Press pp.136–159.

ONS (2000) *Neighbourhood Statistics: Isle of Wight*, http://www.neighbourhood.statistics.gov.uk/tables/eng/TableViewer/wdsview/, accessed 8th October 2002.

Osler, A. (2005) *Teachers, Human Rights and Diversity*, Stoke on Trent: Trentham.

Osler, A. and Starkey, H. (2001) Citizenship education and national identities in France and England: inclusive or exclusive? *Oxford Review of Education*, Vol. 27(2), pp.287–305.

Osler, A. and Starkey, H. (2003) Learning for cosmopolitan citizenship: theoretical debates and young people's experiences, *Educational Review*, Vol. 55(3), pp.243–254.

Osler, A. and Starkey, H. (2005a) *Study on the Advances in Civic Education in Education Systems: Good Practices in Industrialized Countries*, Geneva: International Bureau of Education, UNESCO.

Osler, A. and Starkey, H. (2005b) *Changing Citizenship: Democracy and Inclusion in Education*, Maidenhead: Open University Press.

O'Toole, T. (2003) Engaging with young people's conceptions of the political, *Children's Geographies*, Vol. 1(1), pp.71–90.

Oulton, C., Day, V., Dillon, J. and Grace, M. (2004) Controversial issues – teachers' attitudes and practices in the context of citizenship education, *Oxford Review of Education*, Vol. 30(4), pp.489–507.

Owen, D. (1996) Civics and citizenship: dilemmas and opportunities for the young active citizen, *Youth Studies Australia*, Vol. 15(1), pp.20–23.

Pain, R. (2003) Youth, age and the representation of fear, *Capital and Class*, Vol. 80, Summer, pp.151–171.

Painter, J. and Philo, C. (1995) Spaces of citizenship: an introduction, *Political Geography*, Vol. 14(2), pp.107–120.

Park, P. (1999) People, knowledge, and change in participatory research, *Management Learning*, Vol. 30(2), pp.141–157.

PDHRE (2000) *Human Rights, Children and Youth*, http://www.pdhre.org/rights/children.html, accessed 10th June 2000.

Philo, C. (1997) *War and Peace in the Social Geography of Children*, Paper delivered at Meeting of the ESRC 'Children 5–16' Programme, University of Keele, 17th March.

Philo, C. (2003) 'To go back up the side hill': memories, imaginations and reveries of childhood, *Children's Geographies*, Vol. 1(1), pp.7–23.

Phipps, C. (2003) Children of the Revolution, *The Guardian*, 22nd March.

Piche, D. (1981) The spontaneous geography of the urban child, in Herbert, D.T. and Johnston, R.J. (eds) *Geography and the Urban Environment: Progress in Research and Applications*, Vol. 6, Chichester: John Wiley, pp.229–256.

Pilcher, J. (1995) *Age and Generation in Modern Britain*, Oxford: OUP.

Pretty, J. (1998) *The Living Land*, London: Earthscan.

Price, D. (2000) Boys win court case in fight for play area, *The Independent*, 20th September, p.4.

Probert, S. (2001) Listen as the young ones voice important opinions, *The Birmingham Post*, 5th October, p.3.

Prout, A. (2000) Children's participation: control and self-realisation in British late modernity, *Children & Society*, Vol. 14, pp.304–315.

Putnam, R.D., (2000) *Bowling Alone: The Collapse and Revival of American Community*, New York: Simon and Schuster.

QCA (1998) *Education for Citizenship and the Teaching of Democracy in Schools: Final Report of the Advisory Group on Citizenship*, 22nd September, London: QCA.

QCA (2000) *Citizenship: The National Curriculum for England – Key Stages 3–4*, London: QCA.

RBA (2002) *Are Young People Being Heard?* Leeds: RBA.

Reay, D. and Lucey, H. (2000) 'I don't really like it here but I don't want to be any-where else': children and inner city council estates, *Antipode*, Vol. 32(4), pp.410–428.

Relph, E. (1976) *Place and Placelessness*, London: Pion.

Richardson, A. (1990) *Talking about Commitment: The Views of Young People on Citizenship and Volunteering*, London: SCPR.

Roche, J. (1999) Children: rights, participation and citizenship, *Childhood*, Vol. 6(4), pp.475–493.

Roker, D., Player, K. and Coleman, J. (1999) Young people's voluntary and cam-paigning activities as sources of political education, *Oxford Review of Education*, Vol. 25(1/2), pp.185–198.

Rutland, E. (2002) Wight 2B Heard, *Wight Insight*, Issue 46, May, p.23.

Salvadori, I. (2001) 'Remove a fence, invite chaos': children as active agents of change, *Local Environment*, Vol. 6(1), pp.87–91.

Sangha, B. (2001) *Working Children as Protagonists*, http://www.workingchild.org/prota.htm, accessed 21st January 2001.

Schapiro, T. (1999) What is a child? *Ethics*, July, Vol. 109(4), pp.715–741.

SchNEWS (2004) Minors strike, in SchNEWS (2004) *ScNEWS at Ten*, London: SchNEWS.

Sharp, J.P., Routledge, P., Philo C. and Paddison R. (2000) *Entanglements of Power: Geographies of Domination/Resistance*, London: Routledge.

Sharp, L. (2002) Public participation and policy: unpacking connections in one UK Local Agenda 21, *Local Environment*, Vol. 7(1), pp.7–22.

Shurmer-Smith, P. (2000) Hélène Cixous, in Crang, M. and Thrift, N. (eds) *Thinking Space*, London: Routledge, pp.154–166.

Sibley, D. (1991) Children's geographies: some problems of representation, *Area*, Vol. 23(3), pp.269–270.

Sibley, D. (1995) *Geographies of Exclusion: Society and Difference in the West*, London: Routledge.

Sibley, D. (1999) Creating geographies of difference, in Massey, D., Allen, J. and Sarre, P. (eds) *Human Geography Today*, Cambridge: Polity, pp.115–128.

Skelton, T. (2000) 'Nothing to do, nowhere to go?': teenage girls and 'public' space in the Rhondda Valleys, South Wales, in Holloway, S.L. and Valentine, G. (eds) *Children's Geographies: Playing, Living, Learning*, London: Routledge, pp.80–99.

Skelton, T. (2005) 'The commonwealth games baton arrives in Montserrat': symbols of children's 'citizenship' in a complex political setting, *Children's Geographies*, Vol. 3(3), pp.363–367.

Skelton, T. and Valentine, G. (1998) (eds) *Cool Places: Geographies of Youth Cultures*, London: Routledge.

Smith, L.T., Smith, G.H., Boler, M., Kempton, M., Ormond, A., Chueh, H-C. and Waetford, R. (2002) 'Do you guys hate Aucklanders too?' Youth: voicing difference from the rural heartland, *Journal of Rural Studies*, 18, pp.169–178.

Soysal, Y. (1994) *The Limits of Citizenship*, Chicago: University of Chicago Press.

Staeheli, L.A. and Mitchell, D. (2004) Spaces of public and private: locating politics, in Barnett, C. and Low, M. (eds) *Spaces of Democracy: Geographical Perspectives on Citizenship, Participation and Representation*, London: Sage, pp.147–160.

Stainton-Rogers, R. and Stainton-Rogers, W. (1992) *Stories of Childhood: Shifting Agendas of Childhood Concern*, Hemel Hempstead: Harvester Wheatsheaf.

Steadman, R. (1998) *For the Care of Victims of Torture Celebrate the 50th Anniversary of the Universal Declaration of Human Rights*, London: The Medical Foundation.

Stuart, J. (2000) 'I love spending my mum's money on clothes...' *Independent – The Tuesday Review*, 14th November, p.7.

Sure Start (2002) *Sure Start*, http://www.surestart.gov.uk/aboutsurestart/, accessed 5th December 2002.

Swain, J. (2002) The right stuff: fashioning an identity through clothing in a junior school, *Gender and Education*, Vol. 14(1), pp.53–69.

Taylor, G. (1999) Empowerment, identity and participatory research: using social action research to challenge isolation for deaf and hard of hearing people from minority ethnic communities, *Disability and Society*, Vol. 14(3), pp.369–384.

Taylor, A.S. (2000) The UN Convention on the Rights of the Child: giving children a voice, in Lewis, A. and Lindsay, G. (eds) *Researching Children's Perspectives*, Buckingham: Open University Press, pp.21–33.

Thomas, G. and Hocking, G. (2003) *Other People's Children: Why Their Quality of Life is Our Concern*, London: Demos.

Thomas, N. and O'Kane, C. (1999) Experiences of decision-making in middle childhood: the example of children 'looked after' by Local Authorities, *Childhood*, Vol. 6(3), pp.369–387.

Tooke, J. (2000) Betweenness at work, *Area*, Vol. 32(2), pp.217–224.

Tooley, J. (2000) Foreword, in Flew, A. (2000) *Education for Citizenship*, London: IEA, pp.4–6.

Tranter, P. and Pawson, E. (2001) Children's access to local environments: a case-study of Christchurch, New Zealand, *Local Environment*, Vol. 6(1), pp.27–48.

Travis, A. (2000) Curfew plan gets cold shoulder, *The Guardian*, 7th December, p.13.

Travis, A. (2005) Testing passport to UK citizenship, *The Guardian*, 1st November, http://www.guardian.co.uk/print/0,,5322905-103639,00.html, accessed 21st June 2006.

Tucker, F. (2003) Sameness or difference? Exploring girls' use of recreational space, *Children's Geographies*, Vol. 1(1), pp.111–124.

Tucker, F. and Matthews, M. (2001) 'They don't like girls hanging around there': conflicts over recreational space in rural Northamptonshire, *Area*, Vol. 33(2), pp.161–168.

Turner, L. (2004) From the classroom to the ballot box, *Guardian Education*, 13th January, p.14.

UNICEF (2005) *Special protections: Progress and disparity. Old enough to be a criminal?* http://www.unicef.org /pon97/p56a.htm, accessed 25th February 2005.

United Nations (1990) *Convention on the Rights of the Child*, New York: United Nations.

Valentine, G. (1996) Angels and devils: moral landscapes of childhood, *Environment and Planning D: Society and Space*, Vol. 14, pp.581–599.

Valentine, G. (1999) Being seen and heard? The ethical complexities of working with children and young people at home and at school, *Ethics, Place and Environment*, Vol. 2(2), pp.141–155.

Valentine, G. (2000) Exploring children and young people's narratives of identity, *Geoforum*, 31, pp.257–267.

Valentine, G. (2003) Boundary crossings: transitions from childhood to adulthood, *Children's Geographies*, Vol. 1(1), pp.37–52.

Valentine, G. (2004) *Public Space and the Culture of Childhood*, Aldershot: Ashgate.

Valentine, G. and Holloway, S. (2001) A window on the wider world? Rural children's use of information and communication technologies, *Journal of Rural Studies*, 17, pp.383–394.

Valentine, G., Skelton, T. and Chambers, D. (1998) Cool places: an introduction to youth cultures, in Valentine, G. and Skelton, T. (eds) *Cool Places: Geographies of Youth Cultures*, London: Routledge, pp.1–34.

Vanderbeck, R.M. and Dunkley, C.M. (2003) Young people's narratives of rural-urban difference, *Children's Geographies*, Vol. 1(2), pp.241–259.

Wainwright, M. (2001) Voting early, *Guardian Education*, 29th May, p.7.

Walker, A. (2003) Pupils hurt in the battle of Parliament Square, *Camden New Journal*, 27th March, p.8.

Watt, P. (1998) Going out of town: youth, 'race', and place in the South East of England, *Environment and Planning D: Society and Space*, Vol. 16, pp.687–703.

Watts, M. (2006) Citizenship education revisited: policy, participation and problems, *Pedagogy, Culture & Society*, Vol. 14(1), pp.83–97.

Wellard, S., Tearse, M. and West, A. (1997) *All Together Now: Community Participation for Children and Young People*, London: Save the Children.

Weller, S. (2003) Teach us something useful: contested spaces of teenagers' citizenship, *Space and Polity*, Vol. 7(2), pp.153–172.

Weller, S. (2004a) 'Teenage Citizenship Geographies: Rural Spaces of Exclusion, Education and Creativity, Unpublished PhD thesis, Brunel University.

Weller, S. (2004b) Researching the familiar: age, place and social capital, in Edwards, R. (ed.) *Social Capital in the Field: Researchers' Stories*, Families and Social Capital ESRC Research Group Working Paper No. 10 (London South Bank University, London).

Weller, S. (2006a) Skateboarding alone? Making social capital discourse relevant to teenagers' lives, *Journal of Youth Studies*, Vol. 9 (5), pp.557–574.

Weller, S. (2006b) Situating (young) teenagers in geographies of children and youth, *Children's Geographies*, Vol. 4(1), pp.97–108.

Weller, S. (2006c) Tuning-in to teenagers! The use of radio phone-in discussions in research with young people, *International Journal of Social Research Methodology*, Vol. 9(4), pp.303–315.

Wenger, E. (1998) *Communities of Practice: Learning, Meaning and Identity*, London: CUP.

White, R. and Sutton, A. (2001) Social planning for mall redevelopment: An Australian case-study, *Local Environment*, Vol. 6(1), pp.65–80.

Wight Insight (2001) 'Wight2BHeard' 2001, *Wight Insight*, Issue 38, p.21.

Williamson, J. (2002) The neglect we tolerate, *The Guardian*, 22nd June, pp.22.

Willis, P.E. (2001) Dossing, blagging and wagging: countercultural groups in the school environment, in Giddens, A. (ed.) *Sociology: Introductory Readings*, Cambridge: Polity, pp.209–315.

Willow, C. (2004) Children are ordinary citizens, too, *The Guardian*, 3rd September, p.28.

Wolchover, J. (2002) Today's lesson: citizenship for beginners, *The Independent*, 18th April, pp.4–5.

Woolley, H. (2006) Freedom of the city: contemporary issues and policy influences on children and young people's use of public open space in England, *Children's Geographies*, Vol. 4(1), pp.45–60.

Wragg, T. (2002) How will schools tackle the challenge of turning our students into citizens? *Guardian Education*, 6th August, p.5.

Wyn, J. and White, R. (1997) *Rethinking Youth*, London: Sage.

Wyness, M. (1999) Childhood, agency and educational reform, *Childhood*, Vol. 6(3), pp.353–369.

Wyness, M.G. (2000) *Contesting Childhood*, London: Falmer Press.

Wyness, M. (2003) Children's space and interests: constructing an agenda for student voice, *Children's Geographies*, Vol. 1(2), pp.223–239.

Yin, R.K. (1989) *Case Study Research: Design and Methods*, London: Sage.

Young, L. and Barrett, H. (2001) Issues of access and identity, *Childhood*, Vol. 8(3), pp.383–395.

Index

active citizens 2–3, 43, 84, 115, 131–2, 139, 163–4, 168, 171–2; active citizenship 1–2, 24, 29, 49, 54–5, 58–9, 69, 72–3, 82, 92, 96, 100, 112, 131, 133, 156, 163–8
advisory group 49, 53–8
advocacy geographers 132, 161
agency 6, 32, 39, 45, 57, 89, 94–6, 108, 112, 116, 118, 130, 154; active agents 13, 40
Aitken, Stuart 6, 13
alcohol 14, 65, 74, 78
ambiguity 13–14
anti-social behaviour 15, 48, 51–2, 70, 143
apathy 1, 24, 28, 49, 51, 54, 56, 70, 99, 164–5; teenage 2, 21, 33–5, 48, 51–2, 99, 108, 118, 130–1, 153–6, 164–5, 167–8, 170
Aries, Philippe 9–11

belonging 23–4, 38, 41, 46, 58, 65, 69, 100, 102, 123–7, 133–6, 139, 142, 146, 159–60, 168–70
betweenness 9, 13–14, 140, 164
bike: ramp 117–18; shed 114–16
break-time 89–96
Britain 1, 31, 51, 59
British citizens 22, 36, 159; britishness 32, 59
bus: 'busie' – 113–14, 116, 149; shelter 101–102

campaign 1–2, 27, 34, 51, 80–1, 99, 106, 112, 118–20, 131, 164, 168
caretaker thesis 42

childhood 2, 7, 9–10, 13–15, 30–2, 56–7, 73, 165; apollonian and dionysian 10; 'national' 32
child liberation standpoint 42
Children Act 1989 44
children-centred research 4–7, 18, 132, 163
children's geographies 3–7; 13, 171
citizenship 1, 16, 21–47, 57–9 68, 94, 97, 109–10, 112, 123, 161,164–5, 170; cosmopolitan approach 3, 35–9, 47, 59–60, 69–71, 99–131, 162–3, 165, 171; cumulative notion 3, 97, 162, 166; fluid notion 36, 40, 47, 97, 100, 109–10, 123, 127, 131, 136, 162–3, 165, 167; formation 46; inclusive and exclusive aspects 8, 38–40, 43, 59, 71, 133, 136, 159, 171; meaningful inclusion 46–7, 86, 97, 131–2, 150–4, 159, 170; multiple notions 36, 39, 59, 130–1, 171; radical citizenship 36, 39, 58, 116, 124, 126, 130–1, 165, 167–8, 171–2; in schools 48–98, 166–7; spaces of citizenship 3, 8, 23–4, 32, 36, 38–9, 46–7, 60, 67–68, 81, 88–131, 133, 148, 151, 159, 162–3, 168–9, 171–2; teenagers' problematic relationship 8, 21, 24, 29–35, 41, 46–8, 57–9, 76, 102, 117, 123, 145, 160, 164, 166; and work 31–2, 40, 164
citizenship education 1, 2, 28, 31–2, 34, 37, 48–82, 86, 162–163, 165–167; Citizenship Order 49,